Non-Medical Prescribing

This accessible textbook provides a comprehensive resource for healthcare students and professional students studying non-medical prescribing, taking into account the Royal Pharmaceutical Society (RPS) competency framework for non-medical prescribing.

Non-Medical Prescribing: A Course Companion includes chapters on the context of non-medical prescribing; pharmacology; professional, legal and ethical issues; psychological influences; working in multidisciplinary teams; working with patients with complex conditions and co-morbidities; understanding antibiotics and resistances; prescription writing; and the role of non-medical prescribing leads. Each chapter acts as a self-contained study module, with key facts and areas highlighted, illustrative clinical cases to link learning to practice, and a self-test quiz.

Designed for professionals from a range of non-medical disciplines including nursing, midwifery, pharmacy, physiotherapy and occupational therapy, this book can be used at both pre- and post-registration level.

Alison Pooler is a senior lecturer in the School of Medicine at Keele University. She developed the non-medical prescribing programmes within the School of Nursing and Midwifery at Keele before moving over to work within medicine. She also undertook the role of a Nursing Midwifery Council (NMC) reviewer for non-medical prescribing programmes for a number of years and has completed consultancy work across the UK for other higher education institutes (HEIs) around non-medical prescribing curriculum and standards. A nurse practitioner by background, she graduated from Edinburgh University in 1992 with her nursing degree and worked in many acute areas, finally specializing in respiratory medicine where she worked as a V300 prescriber for a number of years before moving into academia in 2008.

Non-Medical Prescribing
A Course Companion

Edited by Alison Pooler

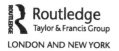

Routledge
Taylor & Francis Group

LONDON AND NEW YORK

First published 2021
by Routledge
2 Park Square, Milton Park, Abingdon, Oxon OX14 4RN

and by Routledge
52 Vanderbilt Avenue, New York, NY 10017

Routledge is an imprint of the Taylor & Francis Group, an informa business

British Library Cataloguing-in-Publication Data
A catalogue record for this book is available from the British Library

Library of Congress Cataloging-in-Publication Data
Names: Pooler, Alison, editor.
Title: Non-medical prescribing: a course companion /
edited by Alison Pooler.
Description: Milton Park, Abingdon, Oxon; New York, NY:
Routledge, 2021. | Includes bibliographical references and index.
Identifiers: LCCN 2020034915 (print) | LCCN 2020034916 (ebook) |
ISBN 9780367281311 (hardback) | ISBN 9780367281342 (paperback) |
ISBN 9780429299827 (ebook)
Subjects: LCSH: Drugs—Prescribing. | Nurses—Prescription privileges. |
Nurse practitioners--Prescription privileges.
Classification: LCC RM138 .N66 2021 (print) |
LCC RM138 (ebook) | DDC 615.1—dc23
LC record available at https://lccn.loc.gov/2020034915
LC ebook record available at https://lccn.loc.gov/2020034916

ISBN: 978-0-367-28131-1 (hbk)
ISBN: 978-0-367-28134-2 (pbk)
ISBN: 978-0-429-29982-7 (ebk)

Typeset in Bembo
by codeMantra

Contents

List of figures   vii
List of tables   viii
List of contributors   ix
Preface   xi

**1 Introduction and development of
    non-medical prescribing**   1
ALISON POOLER

**2 Pharmacology, drug interactions and
    adverse reactions**   15
ALISON POOLER

**3 Prescribing in co-morbidities and
    individual differences**   40
ALISON POOLER

4 Clinical decision-making and assessment   68
ERICA SMITH AND NATALIE RUSCOE

**5 Legal, professional, policy and ethical aspects
    of prescribing**   82
NATALIE RUSCOE AND ERICA SMITH

CONTENTS

6 Psychological influences and issues of concordance   102

ALISON POOLER

7 The public health context of prescribing   115

ALISON POOLER

8 Prescription writing   126

ALISON POOLER

9 The NMP leads and the multidisciplinary team in prescribing   136

ALISON POOLER AND TRACY HALL

Afterword: closing comments – the future of non-medical prescribing   147

ALISON POOLER

Index   149

Figures

1.1 RPS Competency Framework for All Prescribers (2016)   11
2.1 Dosing to maintain a therapeutic level of a drug   26
4.1 Focus of consultations   70
5.1 Accountability responsibilities   83
8.1 Example of an FP10 prescription chart   133

Tables

1.1	Example CMP	8
3.1	Drugs that should be avoided during early pregnancy (due to high risk of causing abortion)	63
5.1	Current non-medical prescribers	87
5.2	Drugs schedules, Misuse of Drugs Regulations, 2001	88
8.1	Abbreviations commonly used when writing prescriptions	130

Contributors

Tracey Hall qualified as an registered general nurse (RGN) in 1987 in North Staffordshire and worked as a Staff Nurse within acute medicine and surgical areas before moving to community nursing in 1996. She qualified as a district nurse (DN) in 2000 and have worked in various areas within District Nursing; in 2004, she set up the Community Matron service. From 2004 to 2007, Tracey was the nurse representative on the Professional Executive Committee (PEC) of the primary care trust (PCT) whereby she was able to influence the decisions being made by the organisation. Tracey became a Queens Nurse in 2007 and joined the Nurse Prescribers Advisory Group of the British national formulary (BNF) shortly after before being asked to join the Joint Formulary Committee of the BNF. Tracey is an Editorial Board Member of Midlands Medicine. She has been the Non-Medical Prescribing Lead for the Trust since 2010.

Alison Pooler graduated from Edinburgh University with her nursing degree in 1992. Since then, she has worked mainly in the acute sector in intensive care, trauma and acute medicine. Eventually specialising in respiratory medicine, she moved over the academia in 2008 to work at Keele University in the School of Nursing and Midwifery and then in the School of Medicine. She developed and led the non-medical prescribing programmes for nine years, providing innovative ways of learning and teaching for the students. She was also a quality assurance

(QA) reviewer for the nursing and midwifery council (NMC) for non-medical prescribing programmes.

Natalie Ruscoe currently works as a Lecturer in Nursing at Keele University's School of Nursing and Midwifery. Natalie's role includes co-leading the Non-Medical Prescribing Module, and she is also the Award Lead for the MSc Advanced Clinical Practice. Natalie is a V300 prescriber and has remained in clinical practice on a part-time basis as an Advanced Nurse Practitioner in the Emergency Department at Royal Stoke University Hospital.

Erica Smith is a Royal College of Emergency Medicine (RCEM) credentialed adult Advanced Clinical Practitioner who works full-time at the Emergency Department of the Royal Stoke University Hospital (University Hospitals of North Midlands NHS Trust). Erica has been an independent non-medical prescriber since 2014 and also guest lecturer at Keele University on the health assessment module.

Preface

Non-medical prescribing is an extended area of clinical practice for many nurses and allied health professionals. Its implementation has grown considerably over the past two decades with more health professionals gaining the legislation to be allowed to undertake this training to enhance their scope of practice and develop more effective services for patients.

The non-medical prescribing course is intense and challenging for many who undertake them. This short companion book summarises and provides the basic information for each of the areas covered in these courses. It provides a grounding on which to develop knowledge further but is not overwhelming as other books with proving too much detail at once.

1 Introduction and development of non-medical prescribing

Alison Pooler

Introduction

Prescribing of medication is commonplace in the modern healthcare system for the treatment and management of conditions. Primarily only within the realm of doctor and dentists, over the past 25 years it has been expanded to other specially trained healthcare professionals to improve patient access to services and improved outcomes for patients.

This chapter gives an overview of the development of non-medical prescribing and the different modes within this concept of prescribing.

Learning objectives

By the end of this chapter, you should be able to

- Have an understanding of the development of non-medical prescribing.
- Appreciate the legislative processes which have occurred to provide the access of non-medical prescribing to the range of healthcare professionals that have permission today.
- Appreciate the impact that this development in access for non-medical prescribing across a range of healthcare professionals has had on patients.
- Understand the different modes of non-medical prescribing.
- Have an understanding of the Royal Pharmaceutical Society (RPS) prescribing framework and its central role in non-medical prescribing.

What is non-medical prescribing?

This is a term used to describe any prescribing of medications undertaken by a health professional, who is not a doctor or dentist. It concerns any medications prescribed by that healthcare professional for conditions and diseases within the field of expertise or that professional.

Why was non-medical prescribing introduced?

There have been significant advances in the United Kingdom over the past 25 years with regard to the prescribing of medications by nurses and other healthcare professionals, who are not doctors nor dentists. The concept of non-medical prescribing was first proposed in 1986 by the Cumberledge Report (DHSS, 1986), which was a review of the care given to people in their own homes by health visitors and district nurses. From this report, it was suggested that access to treatment could be enhanced for people if these community nurses could prescribe. It was also highlighted that use of resources would also be more efficient in terms of healthcare professionals time.

This proposed prescribing activity, however, was from a defined list of items, such as wound dressings and ointments, which were commonly required items for everyday nursing care. From this review, it was also disclosed that often general practitioners (GPs) were signing prescriptions for such items, despite the assessment being done by the community nurses. This not only resulted in wasted hours for both GPs and community nurses but was also not recommended prescribing practice, where assessment of the patient was not carried out by the professional signing the prescription (DH, 1989).

The recommendations from the Cumberledge Report (DHSS, 1986) were then reviewed and developed in the Crown Report in 1989 (DH, 1989). In 1992 legislation was passed to allow community nurses (district nurses and health visitors) to prescribe from an "Extended Formulary for Nurse Prescribers", within the context of a care plan (DHSS, 1992). Pilot areas carried out this new initiative before it was rolled out across the United Kingdom.

In 1999 the second Crown Report (DH, 1999) was released following an extensive review of prescribing, supply and administration of medicines. This review highlighted the need for development of prescribing rights of nurses, due to changes in clinical practice and the developing roles of healthcare professionals from all disciplines. It was felt that there was a need for patients to become more involved in their treatment and to improve access to healthcare for them (DH, 1999). The outcome of this second Crown Report (DH, 1999) was that it recommended that other healthcare professionals would be able to undertake application for legislation to allow them to prescribe in specific clinical areas, which would improve access and effectiveness of healthcare to patients, whilst still ensuring standards of care and safety. The report also recommended the expansion of independent prescribing rights to other nurses to allow more flexibility and autonomy. This meant that nurses were able to prescribe all medicines not only from the original Extended Formulary but also from Pharmacy (P) and general sales (GS) lists, plus certain prescription-only medicines (POM). This was allowed to take place within a supervised framework of practice, which was originally called dependent prescribing, which was later changed to supplementary prescribing, which is a voluntary partnership between an independent and a supplementary prescriber, to implement an agreed patient-specific clinical management plan (CMP) (with the patient's agreement) and to enable prescribing for a specific medical condition or health need affecting the patient (MCA, 2002).

Over the following years up to 2002, supplementary prescribing rights were extended out to other healthcare professionals such as pharmacists (DH, 2001, 2005; MCA, 2002). This was followed in 2005 with the extension to physiotherapists and podiatrists (DH, 2005). In 2006, it was announced that any qualified Extended Formulary nurse prescribers would be able to prescribe any licensed medicine for any medical condition, plus some controlled drugs for specific conditions, as independent prescribers and the Extended Formulary would cease. In independent prescribing, the practitioner is responsible and accountable for the assessment of patients with undiagnosed or diagnosed conditions. If the practitioner is a doctor, then they are also responsible for decisions about the clinical management required, including prescribing (DH, 2005; MHRA, 2005).

The NMC (Nursing and Midwifery Council) also stated that these extended prescribing rights would always be within the individual nurses' area of competence, to ensure parity with the NMC code of professional practice (NMC, 2018). Despite opposition from many within the medical profession, many nurses underwent the required training to undertake this clinical role. For many this formed part of an overall expansion and development of their clinical roles with nurses becoming more autonomous practitioners leading clinical services. Pharmacists quickly followed suit in this role development. Prescribing rights to other healthcare professionals started to cascade, and in 2005 the Department of Health permitted the introduction of supplementary prescribing for physiotherapists and podiatrists (DH, 2005). This was followed in 2007 by optometrists being able to become independent prescribers (DH, 2007) and then in 2013 by physiotherapists and podiatrists also being independent prescribers (DH, 2013). In 2016 NHS England announced new legislation which would allow therapeutic radiographers to become independent prescribers and dieticians to become supplementary prescribers (NHS England, 2016). So the expansion of prescribing rights to a range of healthcare professionals was expanding quickly. This followed ongoing development and expansion of health professional roles to increase autonomy and facilitate service development to meet the needs of a modern healthcare system in the United Kingdom. The most recent legislation (May, 2018) has now expanded these independent prescribing rights to paramedics who work at an autonomous level as a consultant paramedic, most of which work off the ambulances and in primary care and emergency centres.

Impact of non-medical prescribing

With any new development in the healthcare system, time is required for practices to be evaluated and thus allow the generation of evidence based to support practice Any initiative can also be evaluated from various perspectives to gain a holistic view; thus, in this instance it includes the non-medical prescribers (NMPs) themselves, stakeholders, other health professionals and patients.

Staff training to become prescribers felt, and still feel, that the programmes were challenging but provided them with the knowledge and skills to be able to prescribe safely, taking many perspectives into account during their patient encounters (Green et al., 2009; Latter et al., 2010; Meade et al., 2001). Once qualified NMPs have reported increased job satisfaction and self-confident, and being able to prescribe has enabled more effective use of their skills to improve patient outcomes as well as having a positive impact on the relationships they had with their patients and their families (Courtenay & Berry, 2007; George et al., 2007; Watterson et al., 2009). However, they have also reported the increased pressure and workload that prescribing duties brought (Watterson et al., 2009). NMPs and doctors across both primary and secondary care reported that they felt that patients accessing an NMP received higher quality care, with more choice and convenience, often due to increased accessibility and longer consulting times which were available (Courtenay & Berry, 2007; George et al., 2007; Latter et al., 2010; Stewart et al., 2009). Medical staff reported that working with NMPs also increased team working effectiveness, efficiency and positive relations within the team. Often it resulted in a reduction in their workload and freed up time to spend with more complex or acute cases (Stewart et al., 2009; Watterson et al., 2009). These effects were seen once time had been spent supporting the NMPs during their initial time following qualification, but it was felt to be time well spent with longer term gains for all (Hacking & Taylor, 2010; Watterson et al., 2009).

Patient feedback illustrated that they have more efficient access to healthcare with more flexibility to appointments. This was especially so in long-term conditions such as diabetes, asthma and dermatology. Patients reported improved continuity of care and appreciated consultations which were longer and perceived to be more caring (Courtenay et al., 2011; Stenner et.al., 2011). Patients also felt more in control of their conditions and understood their medications better since seeing the NMP (Latter et al., 2010). This positive feedback was all despite initial concerns from patients about seeing a nurse rather than a doctor (Latter et al., 2010; Stewart et al., 2008; Weeks et al., 2016).

Review of clinical practice has revealed that all nurse and pharmacist NMPs were making appropriate and safe decisions around their prescribing practice, despite initial concerns about the depth of pharmacological knowledge of nurses and physical assessment skills of pharmacists (Latter et al., 2012; Naughton et al., 2013). There have, however, been some concerns viewed around the potential risks in the more vulnerable groups such as the elderly, breastfeeding mothers and patients with complex clinical conditions, but these concerns have not resulted or been shown to be apparent in review of clinical practice to date (Naughton et al., 2013). Prescribing errors are always a course for concern for any prescriber and are commonplace for doctors in secondary care settings. Evidence base suggests that there is 7% of all prescriptions are affected by prescribing errors in secondary care written by doctors, affecting 50% of all hospital admissions (Lewis et al., 2009). However, there is a lack of data for non-medical prescribing errors. Ashcroft et al. (2015) aimed to compare the prevalence of prescribing errors in secondary care between first year doctors, senior doctors and NMPs, but this was not possible as the number of prescriptions completed by the NMPs was less than 1% of the total, so no comparisons could be made.

There is some evidence to suggest that nurse NMPs are safe (Latter et al., 2010), and there appears to be few differences between nurses and doctors with regard to the type and dose of medications prescribed in a given clinical area (Gielen et al., 2014). However, there is still a need for more research to generate a more sustainable evidence base to support this practice and evaluate the true impact of non-medical prescribing across all healthcare professionals involved.

Data from 2016 showed that there were around 37,000 nurses qualified as independent prescribers in the United Kingdom (DH, 2016), representing 5% of the nursing workforce and practicing in a wide variety of clinical areas (Courtenay, 2017; Latter et al., 2018). Over 50% had a qualification at master's level, majority had more than five years of clinical experience before completing the prescribing course and they all prescribed independently (Courtenay,

2017). With the expansion of prescribing rights to other healthcare professionals, this number will rise dramatically, thus developing a sustainable workforce fit for a new modern NHS (DHSC, 2015).

Modes of non-medical prescribing

There are two modes of non-medical prescribing: independent and supplementary prescribing. Each has its different responsibilities attached to it, and healthcare professionals have to be aware of these and also work within their own professional codes of conduct.

Supplementary prescribing

This was formerly known as dependent prescribing and is a voluntary partnership between an independent prescriber, who has to be a doctor, and a supplementary prescriber. The aim is to implement an agreed patient-specific CMP with the patient's agreement for a medical condition or a health need (DH, 2006).

The independent prescriber in this prescribing relationship, who must be a doctor, will discuss with the supplementary prescriber which patients may benefit from this mode of prescribing and also what medications to be included in the CMP. The independent prescriber also holds the overall responsibility for the patient's care as they are the ones who make the diagnosis and set the parameters for the CMP. The supplementary prescriber has discretion on the doses and frequency of the medicines within the CMP once developed but must always report back to the independent prescriber within given parameters set for the patient's condition and also time periods for review. It must, however, be remembered that the patient themselves are integral to this prescribing partnership, and all discussion should also involve them for their consent to have their medications prescribed in this format.

CMPs are integral to the mode of supplementary prescribing, without which the prescribing would not occur. They are an agreed defined plan of treatment for a named patient which sets the legal boundaries for the medication and the parameters of prescribing responsibility for the supplementary prescriber. So in essence it is legal framework for a named patient and a specified condition. Once devised, the supplementary prescriber can prescribe anything from that CMP; this is why it is important to have a voluntary agreement between the independent, supplement prescriber and the patient for this arrangement to occur. The supplementary prescriber must still prescribe within their area of competence and ensure all parties in this partnership have access to the CMP which should be held within the multidisciplinary notes for shared access with other healthcare professionals involved in the care of the individual patient.

There are many variations of CMPs in circulation, but as long as they include the minimum information as set out by the Department of Health (2006), they are appropriate to use. Table 1.1 is an example of a CMP.

Table 1.1 Example CMP

Name of patient	*Patient medication sensitivities/allergies*		
Patient identification, e.g. ID number, date of birth:			
Independent prescriber(s):	Supplementary prescriber(s)		
Condition(s) to be treated	Aim of treatment		
Past medical history	Current medication		
Medicines that may be prescribed by SP:			
Preparation	Indication	Dose schedule	Specific indications for referral back to the IP
Guidelines or protocols supporting clinical management plan:			
Frequency of review and monitoring by:			
Supplementary prescriber OR Supplementary prescriber and independent prescriber			
Process for reporting ADRs:			
Shared record to be used by IP and SP:			
Agreed by independent prescriber(s)	Date	Agreed by supplementary prescriber(s)	Date	Date agreed with patient/carer

Notes: SP = supplementary prescriber; IP= independent prescriber; ADRs = adverse drug reactions

There are no legal restrictions on the conditions which can be treated or on what can be prescribed as a result of the CMP. However, where possible, the CMP should state national or locally agreed guidelines. Medications should be prescribed using their generic names except where not clinically indicated, for example in the case of a drug with a specific bioavailability or where the product does not have an approved generic name.

Supplementary prescribing is best used in a number of situations, such as the following:

- When the patient's condition requires treatment with unlicensed medications
- When medications are required which are going to be used outside of their product licence, for example smoking cessation patches for teenagers
- For controlled drugs which may not be permitted to be prescribed by the independent NMP prescriber, maybe because of local policy as well as national policy
- For the management of complex conditions where shared care is a necessity
- For the new NMP to gain confidence in prescribing, this is common in primary care where practice nurses may take on this role and find using a CMP as a way of building their confidence when running nurse-led clinics where complex patients may be reviewed

Independent prescribing

Independent prescribers are practitioners who are responsible and accountable for the assessment of patients with previously undiagnosed or diagnosed health conditions. They are also responsible for the decisions about the clinical management required of these conditions, which includes prescribing of medications. It is recommended that when prescribing generic names are used, except where this would not be clinically appropriate, for example when prescribing a salbutamol inhaler which has to fit in a Volumatic spacer, or when a patient responds better clinically to a certain brand-named product, or where there is no approved non-proprietary name.

All independent prescribers must work within their own level of competence and expertise, according to their professional code of conduct. Healthcare professionals who can train to become NMPs includes (at the time of writing January 2020) nurses, midwives, physiotherapists, podiatrists, optometrists, therapeutic radiographers and paramedics (who work as a consultant practitioner within clinical practice).

To become an NMP, either independent and/or supplementary, healthcare professionals who are allowed to undertake such training have to access and complete an approved training programme which is validated by the professional bodies of the NMC, healthcare professions council (HCPC) or general pharmaceutical council (GPhC). Central to these training programmes is the Royal Pharmaceutical Society's (RPS) Competency Framework for All Prescribers (RPS, 2016). This framework outlines a clear set of competencies which have to be met and maintained post initial training. The competencies are made up of knowledge, skills and personal traits that are expected of safe and effective prescribers.

The RPS's Competency Framework for All Prescribers

This is a generic framework which relates to both independent and supplementary prescribing roles, within any professional background. Its purpose is to ensure a suitable standard and bench mark of quality for prescribing and that safety is maintained. Professional accountability is a central concept of the framework, and the whole framework relates not only to the prescribing of medications but also to advice about medications and ongoing management of patients using medications (RPS, 2016).

The framework outlines what good prescribing practice should resemble, and within it there are ten competencies divided into two broad domains (see Figure 1.1).

Each of these competences is embedded into all non-medical prescribing course in the United Kingdom to guide the curriculum being taught and examined. They can also be used for annual

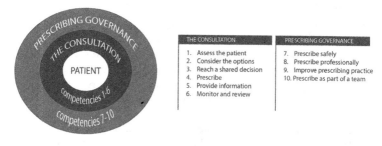

The Consultation
1. Assess the patient
2. Consider the options
3. Reach a shared decision
4. Prescribe
5. Provide information
6. Monitor and review

Prescribing Governance
7. Prescribe safely
8. Prescribe professionally
9. Improve prescribing practice
10. Prescribe as part of a team

Figure 1.1 RPS Competency Framework for All Prescribers (2016).

appraisals to ensure standards in prescribing practice are maintained post qualification and to aid the development of target for continued professional development.

Self-assessment test

1   What was the outcome of the Cumberlege Report?
2   What was the outcome of the second Crown Report for non-medical prescribing?
3   What is the role of the independent and supplementary prescribers in the supplementary prescribing arrangement?
4   What is central to the supplementary prescribing mode of non-medical prescribing?
5   What are the differences between independent and supplementary prescribing roles?
6   What is the relevance of the RPS framework to non-medical prescribing?

Reflective exercise

You have now red through this chapter and studied its contents, so it is time to reflect on what you have learnt and how it can be applied to your own professional practice. Think about your own are of potential prescribing or current prescribing; how do you see your role as an NMP developing and how will the RPS framework feature in this development?

References

Ashcroft, D.M., Lewis, P.J., Tully, M.P., Farrangher, T.M., Taylor, D., Wass, V., Williams S.D., & Dornan, T. (2015). Prevalence, nature, severity and risk factors for prescribing errors in hospital in patients. Prospective study in 20 UK hospitals. *Drug Safety*. 38, 833–843.

Courtenay, M., & Berry, D. (2007). Comparing nurses and doctors' views of nurse prescribing; a questionnaire survey. *Nurse Prescribing*. 5, 205–210.

Courtenay, M., Coey, N., Steener, K., Lawton, S., & Peters, J. (2011). Patients views of nurse prescribing; effects on care, concordance and medicine taking. *The British Journal of Dermatology*. 164, 396–401.

Courtenay, M., Khanfer, R., & Harries-Huntly, G. (2017). Overview of the uptake and implementation of non-medical prescribing in Wales; a national survey. *BMJ Open*. 7(9), 015313.

Department of Health (DH). (1989). *Report of the advisory group on nurse prescribing (Crown Report)*. London: DH.

Department of Health (DH). (1992). *Medicinal products; prescribing by nurse act*. London: DH.

Department of Health (DH). (1999). *Review of prescribing, supply and administration of medicines, Final Report (Crown II Report)*. London: DH.

Department of Health (DH). (2001). *Health and social care act*. London: DH.

Department of Health (DH). (2003). *Amendments to the POM amendments order and NHS regulations*. London: DH.

Department of Health (DH). (2005). *Nurse and pharmacist prescribing powers extended*. London: DH.

Department of Health (DH). (2006). *Improving patient's access to medicines; a guide to implementing nurse and pharmacist independent prescribing within the NHS in England*. London: DH.

Department of Health (DH). (2013). *The medicines act 1968 and the human medicines regulations (Amendment) order*. London: DH.

Department of Health and Social Security (DHSS). (1986). *Neighbourhood nursing; a focus of care. Report of the community nursing review*. Cumberledge Report. London: HMSO.

Department of Health and Social Security (DHSS). (2015). *NHS constitution for England*. London: HMSO.

George, J., McCaig, D., Bond, C., Cunningham, J., Diack, H., & Stewart. D. (2007). Benefits and challenges of prescribing training and implementation; perceptions and early experience of RPSGB prescribers. *International Journal of Pharmacy Practice*. 15, 23–30.

Gielen, S.C., Dekker, J., & Francke, A. (2014). The effects of nurse prescribing; a systematic review. *International Journal of Nursing Studies*. 51(-7), 1048–1061.

Green, A., Westwood, O., Smith, P., Peniston-Bird, F., & Holloway, D. (2009). Provision of continued professional development for non-medical prescribers within a South of England Strategic Health Authority; a report on training needs analysis. *Journal of Nursing Management*. 17, 603–614.

Hacking, S., & Taylor, J. (2010). An evaluation of the scope and practice of non-medical prescribing in the North West for NHS NW. Available at https://www.researchgate.net/publication/228406352_An_evaluation_of_the_scope_and_practice_of_Non_Medical_Prescribing_in_the_North_West_For_NHS_North_West

Latter, S., Blenkinsopp, A., Smith, A., Chapman, S., Tinelli, M., & Gerrad, K. (2010). *Evaluation of nurse and pharmacist independent prescribing*. London: DH.

Lewis, P., Darnan, T., Taylor, D., Tully, M., Wass, V., & Ashcroft, D. (2009). Prevalence incidence and nature of prescribing errors in hospital inpatients. *Drug Safety*. 32, 379–389.

Meade, O., Bowskill, D., & Lymm, J. (2011). Pharmacology podcasts, a qualitative study of NMP students' use, perceptions and impact on learning. *BMC Medical Education*. 11, 2.

Medicines and health care Products Regulatory Agency (MHRA). (2005). *Consultation on proposals to introduce independent prescribing by pharmacists MLX 321*. London: MHRA.

Medicines Control Agency (MCA). (2002). *Proposals for supplementary prescribing by nurses and pharmacists and proposed amendments to the prescription only medicines (Human use) Order 1997*. MLX 284. London: MCA.

Naughton, C., Drennan, J., Hyde, A., Allen, D., O'Boyle, K., & Felle, P. (2013). An evaluation of the appropriateness and safety of nurse and midwife prescribing in Ireland. *Journal of Advanced Nursing*. 69, 1478–1488.

NHS England. (2016). *Allied health professions medicines project*. London: NHS. Available at http://www.england.nhs.uk/ourwork/qual-clin-lead/ahp-a/. Accessed 11 February 2020.

Nursing and Midwifery Council (NMC). (2018). *The code*. London: NMC.

Royal Pharmaceutical Society (RPS). (2016). *Competency framework for all prescribers*. London: NICE.

Stenner, K., & Courtenay, M., & Carey, N. (2011). Consultations between nurse prescribers and patients with diabetes in primary care; a qualitative study of patients' views. *International Journal of Nursing Studies*. 48, 37–46.

Stewart, D., George, J., Bond, C., Diack, L., McCaig, D., & Cunningham, S. (2009). Views of pharmacist prescribers, doctors and patients on pharmacists prescribing implementation. *International Journal of Pharmacy Practice*. 17(2), 89–94.

Watterson, A., Turner, F., Coull, A., & Murray I. (2009). *An evaluation of the expansion of nurse prescribing in Scotland (Final Report)*. Edinburgh: Scottish Government in Social Research.

Weeks, G., George, J., MaClure, K., & Stewart, D. (2016). Non medical prescribing versus medical prescribing for acute and chronic disease management in primary and secondary care. *Cochrane Data Base of Systematic Reviews*. 11(11), CD011227.

While, A.E., & Biggs, K.S. (2004). Benefits and challenges of nurse prescribing. *Journal of Advanced Nursing*. 45(6), 559–567.

2 Pharmacology, drug interactions and adverse reactions

Alison Pooler

Introduction

There are an enormous number of drugs available, both with and without a prescription. To be able to understand how drugs work, therefore, is crucial. Contribution to treatment decisions can only be achieved if the individual health professional understands how drugs work and exert their effects on the body and also what affects the body itself exerts on the drugs.

This chapter looks at the science of pharmacology, which encompasses pharmacodynamics and pharmacokinetics. It also looks at the considerations that need to be made around polypharmacy and drug interactions. It will also look at the process of how drugs are licensed to allow appreciation of this process and know where the information supplied in the BNF about each drug comes from.

Learning objectives

By the end of this chapter, students should be able to

- Define the terms "pharmacology", "pharmacodynamics" and "pharmacokinetics"
- Outline the mechanisms by which drugs act
- Describe the four pharmacokinetic processes that a drug undergoes
- Be able to apply knowledge of drug actions in prescribing practice

- Understand how drugs are developed and licensed
- Understand the principles of polypharmacy and the consequences this can have on patients
- Understand and be able to apply ways of reducing the effects of polypharmacy in clinical practice
- Understand the nature of drug interactions and apply the principles to their clinical practice
- Understand how adverse drug reactions are reported

Pharmacology

The term "pharmacology" is a broad term, which includes two defined elements: pharmacodynamics and pharmacokinetics. These concepts outline the actions, mechanisms, uses and adverse effects of drugs and medicines which enter the body and the effects that they have.

Drug names and classification

A drug is any natural substance that alters the physiological state of a living organism. A single drug can have a variety of names and belongs to a variety of different classes. Factors that are used to classify drugs include the following:

- Pharmacotherapeutic actions
- Pharmacological actions
- Molecular actions
- Chemical nature

The generic name of a drug is that which appears in official national formularies. When a drug company's patent expires, the marketing of the drug is open to any number of manufacturers. Although the generic name is retained, the variety of brand names increases as different pharmaceutical companies use different brand names for the same drug. Examples are given as follows:

Generic name = Salbutamol
Brand name(s) = Salamol, Airomir

Generic name = Paracetamol
Brand name = Calpol

Is the patient getting the drug: routes of administration of drugs into the body

Before any pharmacokinetic processes occur, we first need to en-sure that the drug actually gets into the patient. There are many different routes of administration but also formulation of drugs to aid this process for patients given their individual characteristics and circumstances.

Routes of administration for drugs include the following:

* Oral
* Sublingual/buccal
* Parenteral (e.g. subcutaneous (SC), intravenous (IV), intra-muscular (IM))
* Inhalation
* Topical (eye, skin, ears, nasal mucosa)
* Rectal
* Vaginal

What this list illustrates is that in most cases a drug has to be avail-able systemically to produce its effects. But there are a few hurdles to cross before the drug gets into the systemic circulation; for ex-ample when taken orally, the drug has two hurdles to encounter: the intestinal wall and the liver.

Oral: Most drugs are given by this route as it is the most conve-nient. However, some drugs are destroyed by enzymes in the gut via first-pass metabolism (discussed later); therefore, they must be given parenterally.

Sublingual: This is extensively metabolised in the liver so it cannot be given orally (e.g. glycerol trinitrate (GTN)). This is why we give isosorbide mononitrate (ISMN) or isosorbide dinitrate (ISDN), which are ultimately metabolised in the liver to nitric acid the same as GTN (this is to do with the first-pass effect of the liver and will be discussed later). There is also a very efficient capillary blood supply in the mucous membranes of the mouth to aid the absorption of the drug via this route.

Buccal: The advantage, as with sublingual and topical administration, is that first-pass metabolism, which occurs in the liver, is avoided and again also the good capillary blood supply in this area to aid effective drug absorption (e.g. chewing an aspirin when having a myocardial infarction, as buccal absorption occurs).

Intravenous (IV): This route gives direct access to the circulation and bypasses the absorption barriers because this drug is 100% bioavailable in the circulatory system. It is used for rapid effect, for large volumes and for drugs that cause local tissue damage if given by other routes such as hydrocortisone being given intramuscularly.

SC and IM: Drugs in aqueous solutions are usually absorbed fairly rapidly, but absorption can be slowed by formulating the drug as an ester, for example, with depot neuroleptics. For SC and IM, absorption depends greatly on the site of injection and local blood flow.

Inhalation: e.g. for anaesthetics where the lungs act as the route for administration and elimination for the drug or for drugs where a local effect is required, such as inhaled steroids and bronchodilators in asthma and chronic obstructive pulmonary disease (COPD) treatment. The drugs act directly on the receptors. Using the inhalation route for drugs to treat asthma is quicker than using the oral route and also requires smaller doses, for example to compare 100 mcg of salbutamol inhaled to 5 mg of salbutamol liquid, and also the side effects of the liquid format of salbutamol are higher than those of the inhaled salbutamol.

Topical: It can be used for systemic effects (e.g. hormone replacement therapy (HRT) and nicotine replacement therapy (NRT) patches) and also for local effect on the skin such as steroids for eczema. It should always be remembered that although a drug is applied to the skin, it can have systemic effects especially if the drug is lipid soluble.

Eyes: This route can be used for local effects such as infections of the eye or glaucoma. Need to be aware of systemic absorption which can occur; for example beta blocker eye drops can have cardiovascular side effects and also side effects such as bronchoconstriction in asthmatics.

Ears: This route is used for local effects in the ear such as steroid drops for infections or preparations to soften wax within the ear.

Rectal: This route can be used for local effects such as steroid preparation for ulcerative colitis or systemic effects such as nonsteroidal anti-inflammatory drugs (NSAIDs). Absorption following rectal administration is often unreliable but can be useful in patients who are vomiting or unable to take medication by mouth.

Vaginal: This route is mainly used for local effects (e.g. antifungal preparations for *Candida*).

Drug formulation is also an important feature which includes concepts such as tablet size, whether it is a modified release preparation, whether it has an enteric coating and how compressed the material of the tablet is, all of which can affect the rate of absorption. Formulation is also considered in terms of if the drug is a liquid or aerosol and the devise in which these may be available in. A further aspect to be considered in all of these is the ability of the patient to take the actual drug and their concordance with the drug, whether it be less effective due to either intended or unintended compliance with the drug itself.

Pharmacokinetics

There are four processes involved in pharmacokinetics of drugs:

Absorption
Distribution
Metabolism
Excretion

The abbreviation ADME is thus commonly used.

Why do we need to know about ADME?

The knowledge and understanding of how a drug is handled by the body can help us to appreciate the importance of individual variation, to choose an effective regimen of treatment while mini-mising risks and to anticipate problems, for example drug-to-drug interactions, and also to consider the effects of impaired organ functioning and how this can affect the way the drug is handled by the body.

Absorption of oral drugs

There are a number of barriers that a drug taken orally has to pass before reaching the systemic circulation. Firstly, a drug in tablet or capsule form needs to disperse before the process of absorption be-gins. Then, in simple terms, the drug passes through the intestinal wall and enters the portal circulation where it is delivered to the liver. In the liver the drug may be metabolised before it reaches the systemic circulation, known as the first-pass metabolism or the first-pass effect. There are some drugs such as insulin and ben-zyl penicillin, which are completely inactivated by gastric acids and enzymes of first-pass metabolism; hence, these are never taken orally. Drugs are metabolised to varying degrees; hence, why dos-ages of drugs given orally may be higher than those given via other routes such as inhaled or IV to take into account this first-pass metabolism effect. For example, salbutamol is given orally in doses of 5–10 mg and in the inhaled form it is 100 mcg as a starting dose from an inhaler.

Therefore, there are two processes that reduce the amount of drug that reaches the circulation for distribution: crossing the in-testinal wall and the enzyme systems of the liver. The amount of drug that reaches the systemic circulation intact is known as the bioavailability of the drug.

The mechanism of absorption through the intestinal wall usu-ally involves passive transfer at a rate determined by the concentra-tion gradient, the surface area for absorption and the fat solubility of the drug itself. For some drugs, absorption depends on carrier-mediated transport, for example glucose, sodium and potassium, rather than lipid diffusion. Little absorption occurs until the drug enters the small intestine.

Factors that can affect the rate, site and extent of absorption are as follows:

1   Rate of gastric emptying/gastric mobility
2   Particle size and formulation
3   Physiochemical interactions with other drugs and food
    substances
4   Malabsorption states

Rate of gastric emptying/gastric mobility: Drugs acting on cholinergic, opioid or dopaminergic receptors, by slowing down
the gastrointestinal (GI) transit, can affect the rate at which
other drugs are absorbed in the jejunum, which can lead to
failure of a drug to reach its therapeutic plasma level. Drugs
that enhance gastric mobility, for example metoclopramide,
will accelerate the absorption of analgesics such as paracetamol,
which protects their therapeutic effect in situations that lead to
gastric stasis, for example migraine. Such changes do not lead
to changes in bioavailability. Drug absorption occurs mainly
in the upper part of the small intestine, so the speed of gastric
emptying determines the speed at which the drug reaches its
site of absorption. Any changes in the speed will affect the rate
of absorption, for example. In migraine the speed of absorption of analgesics is recued because of reduced gastric mobility
with associated nausea and therefore can be a poor response to
analgesia. This can be counteracted by the administration of
metoclopramide which increases the speed of gastric emptying
and reduces nausea.

Particle size and formulation: Modified-released preparations
allow the dose interval to increase and reduce adverse effects
related to peak concentrations, for example nifedipine. Enteric
coating of tablets allows them to pass through the stomach intact, but the coating breaks down in the higher pH of the small
intestine.

Physiochemical interactions: Reactions such as this in the gut
can prevent (reduce the extent of) absorption, for example tetracycline and calcium, colestyramine and warfarin/digoxin. Food
can also interact with drugs and either enhance or impair the
rate of absorption and their extranet of absorption; for example
eggs impair the absorption of iron and milk impairs the absorption of tetracycline. Most penicillin antibiotics have their speed

of absorption impaired by food, but metoprolol, propranolol and hydralazine, for example, have a faster rate of absorption with food present in the gut. Interactions that can reduce the extent of absorption are easily manageable by spacing doses between different drugs.

Malabsorption states: Conditions such as coeliac, ulcerative colitis and Crohn's disease can affect the absorption of drugs. These effects are not always to slow down the rate of absorption. For example, the absorption of propranolol is increased in patients with coeliac disease and Crohn's disease. Digoxin, however, is absorbed from tablets less well in patients with coeliac disease, radiation-induced enteritis and other GI conditions, either acute or chronic presentations.

Distribution of drugs

The aim of this process is to get the absorbed drug to its site of action. Distribution around the body occurs when the drug reaches the systemic circulation. It must then penetrate the tissues to act. This usually occurs by passive diffusion and well-perfused tissues receive the highest drug concentrations faster; hence, the efficiency of the circulatory system is an important factor. So conditions such as ischaemic heart disease or dehydration, which affect the efficiency of the circulation, can have an impact on the efficiency of the distribution of drugs. Dehydration is an issue due to decreased fluid volume within the body, and decreased blood pressure which can occur, which is a reflection on the flow of blood around the body.

Once in the bloodstream, the drug passes out of the capillaries under a positive concentration gradient in the interstitial fluid until there is equilibrium between plasma and interstitial fluid concentrations. Gradually, as the concentration falls, there is a positive gradient in the interstitial fluid so the reverse happens. With continued, regular dosing, the next dose is absorbed before the previous dose is fully eliminated; thus, a steady-state concentration of drug is reached where rate in equals rate out (the drug has reached approximately five half-lives).

***Tissue distribution*:** Drugs that are not bound to plasma proteins will be distributed to the tissues of the body. The extent of this varies from drug to drug and various factors influence this distribution such as plasma protein binding and availability of specific receptor sites in tissues, which decrease in increasing age and conditions such as infection, region blood flow and renal functioning. Lipid solubility is another factor, and since cell membranes are composed mostly of lipoproteins, lipid-soluble drugs such as anaesthetics distribute quicker than non-lipid-soluble drugs; this is why obesity can have an effect on the distribution of non-lipid-soluble drugs.

***Protein binding*:** When in the circulation many drugs are bound to plasma proteins such as albumin, for example warfarin and globulins (hormones). The proportion of the bound drug is in equilibrium with the "free fraction", which is thus available for systemic distribution. Only the fraction of the drug that is NOT protein bound can bind to cellular receptors, pass across tissue membranes and gain access to cellular enzymes, thus being distributed to body tissues, metabolised and excreted. Changes in protein binding can therefore cause changes in drug distribution (speed and location).

Protein binding can reduce in renal insufficiency where binding to albumin is decreased; referred to as hypalbuminaemia, and occurs for example in pregnancy. It can also occur due to displacement by other drugs, where they compete for receptor sites and the drug with the higher affinity for the receptor site wins. Finally it also occurs in diseases such as infections where glycoprotein is increased or in trauma or post-surgery where again glycoprotein increases. A possible interaction of two drugs that are extensively protein bound, when co-administered, is displacement of some drug from the protein, due to the drugs competing for the same binding sites on protein molecules in plasma and tissues. Displacement results in an increase in the unbound concentration of a drug in plasma. The consequences of such displacement interactions are transient, and an increase in elimination of the unbound fraction occurs, which usually has minimal if any influence on the clinical effects of the drug.

Metabolism

This mostly occurs in the liver but can also occur in the gut, biliary tract and lungs, and the aim is to produce a water-soluble compound that can be excreted in the urine. Metabolism can be divided into two phases of enzymatic reactions:

Phase 1: This involves chemical alteration of the basic structure of the drug by oxidation, reduction or hydrolysis. A group of enzymes known as cytochrome P450 catalyse a variety of oxidative and reductive reactions which break the drugs down into smaller components. These smaller components are then ready for further reactions to occur in phase 2 of drug metabolism. At the end of phase 1, the majority of drugs are broken down into inactive components; however, this is not always the case. For example, morphine components are still active at the end Phase 1, which means they can still exert an effect on the body until metabolism is complete.

Phase 2: During this second phase, the metabolites are made water soluble so that they can be excreted by the kidneys easily. This is achieved via a process of conjugation which involves endogenous compounds in the liver building the metabolites into compounds which are water soluble. For some conjugates excreted in the biliary tract, deconjugation may occur in the large intestine allowing reabsorption of the active drug (called enterohepatic recycling). Deconjugation may also be reduced by broad-spectrum antibiotics, which destroy intestinal bacterial flora, thus not allowing oestrogen to be reabsorbed into the circulation. The effect is reduced blood levels of oestrogen, which can reduce the contraceptive effectiveness being taken by the person.

Drug metabolism has two important effects:

1   To make the drug more hydrophilic, it speeds excretion in the kidneys because the less lipid-soluble metabolites are not readily reabsorbed in the renal tubules.

2   The metabolites are usually less active, with the exception of metabolites of prodrugs, which are active until both phases of metabolism are complete. For example, morphine converts to the metabolite morphine-6-glucuronide which still has active effects until complete metabolism has occurred. There are a

few some drugs however, which are excreted in the urine in an unchanged state from that administered, for example gentamycin; hence, urine levels can be tested for therapeutic reasons.

There are some drugs that are excreted in the urine unchanged, for example gentamycin.

Factors which affect drug metabolism include the following:

- Genetic factors – due to generic variations in pharmacokinetics and pharmacodynamics of drugs and heightened sensitivity to some drugs
- Other drugs and their interactions
- Hepatic blood flow – if the blood flow to the liver is reduced, then this can result in a build-up of metabolites and a reduction in the efficiency of drugs being metabolised; hence, they stay within the circulatory system causing toxic effects
- Liver disease, which has as similar effect as a reduced blood flow to the liver
- Age – metabolism can be impaired due to a decrease in the production of the enzymes required for drug metabolism. This is especially important to consider in the very young and the elderly hence why dosages may be altered.

Excretion

The main route of excretion of drugs is the kidney. Other routes include the lungs, breast milk, sweat, tears, genital secretions, bile and saliva, and a proportion of some drugs are excreted unchanged in the faeces. This represents the unabsorbed fraction of the drug and/or fractions excreted in the bile. As the kidneys are the most important organs of excretion of drugs, substantial changes occur if there is impaired renal function and this will be considered in Chapter 3.

There are three mechanisms for the excretion of drugs in the kidney:

1 Water-soluble compounds via glomerular filtration
2 Lipid-soluble compounds that are reabsorbed in the renal tubules by passive diffusion

3   Weak acids and bases, which are actively secreted in the prox-
    imal tubules, for example penicillin.

Thus, total renal excretion = excretion by filtration + excretion by
secretion − retention by reabsorption.

If an active drug is metabolised mainly to inactive compounds,
renal function will not affect the elimination of the compound
very much. However, if the drug or an active metabolite is excreted unchanged via the kidneys, changes in renal function will
influence its elimination.

Important terms to remember

Half-life

The half-life of a drug is the time taken for the initial concentration of the drug in the blood to fall by half; this gives an indication
of the rate of elimination.

Knowledge of the half-life is used to establish the dose and frequency of dose required to maintain circulating blood levels of the
drug at a therapeutic level (Figure 2.1). This requires an understanding of the metabolism of the drug, as metabolites can also be active
and therefore exert a similar therapeutic effect to that of the administered drug. The half-life is affected by absorption, metabolism

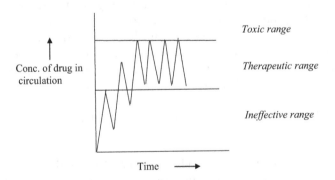

Figure 2.1 Dosing to maintain a therapeutic level of a drug.

and elimination. We need to be aware of this, as this influences how often the drug needs to be administered, for example dosing intervals. The aim of dosing is to produce a stable concentration of the drug in the bloodstream. A drug that is administered regularly is said to reach a "steady state" (concentration); that is, the drug levels within the body stay at a therapeutically effective concentration below toxic levels and above the minimum effective level.

Bioavailability

Before a drug can be effective, it must reach the receptor site in an adequate quantity to produce a response. Drugs given intravenously have a high bioavailability, because they are delivered directly into the bloodstream. Administration via other routes involves processes that reduce the amount of drug available, such as first-pass metabolism for dugs given via the oral route.

Bioavailability is affected by the following:

1   Dose
2   Duration of action (plasma half-life)
3   Route of administration
4   Patient factors, for example disease processes

Pharmacodynamics

In brief, this term refers to how drugs produce their effects on the body and what the drugs do to the body. It refers to the mechanism of action of the drug, the effects of the drug, etc.

How do drugs work?

Drugs work by various mechanisms, which include interacting with the following:

*   Receptors
*   Enzymes
*   Transport systems, for example ion channels and carrier molecules

Interaction with a receptor

A receptor is a protein molecule, which is situated on a cell membrane or within cellular cytoplasm, that is normally activated by transmitters or hormones, for example adrenaline. For each type of receptor, there is a specific group of drugs or endogenous substances (ligands) that are capable of binding to the receptor and thereby producing an effect. An analogy for this is to consider the lock and key action, where the transmitter/hormone is the key that fits the lock. This causes a conformational change in the receptor that initiates a sequence of events, which ultimately produces the effects seen, for example muscle contraction or reduction of inflammation.

Normally, the interaction of a chemical with a receptor triggers a sequence of events involving a second messenger and ultimately results in a biological effect; for example acetylcholine released from motor neuron endings activates receptors in skeletal muscle initiating a sequence of events, which results in contraction of the muscle. Following the release of the natural transmitter, it is inactivated by enzyme degradation or reuptake into the nerve endings. Both modes offer opportunities for drugs to act, for example prevention of enzymatic degradation such as catechol-o-methyltransferase (COMT) inhibitors in Parkinson's disease and selective serotonin reuptake inhibitors (SSRIs) in depression.

Hormones produce their effect by interaction with tissues that possess the necessary specific hormone receptors. Drugs may interact with the endocrine system to inhibit or increase hormone release, for example anti-thyroid drugs and sulphonylureas, respectively. Other drugs interact with hormone receptors which may be activated; for example, steroids and others block the oestrogen receptor antagonists such as tamoxifen.

Other local hormones are released in pathological processes, for example, histamine, serotonin, and prostaglandin. The ability of a drug to combine with one particular type of receptor is called specificity. No drug is truly specific, but many have relatively selective action on one type of receptor. Hence, drugs given to produce a therapeutic effect often exert additional unwanted effects. As an example, consider the range of anticholinergic side effects of procyclidine, given to reduce the cholinergic effects experienced by patients with Parkinson's disease.

The actions of drugs with receptors can be classified as follows:

Agonists: Where the drug mimics the action of the natural chemical/transmitter to produce an appropriate response, for example beta-2 agonists relaxing the smooth muscles in the walls of the airways.

Antagonists: Where they block the action or fit the receptor of the natural chemical/transmitter, but do not activate it, for example beta blockers/H2 antagonists. By preventing this connection, it blocks a response which may be unwanted; for example, anticholinergics such as ipratropium block the M2 receptors in the airway smooth muscles to block the parasympathetic response which would have constructed the smooth muscle and caused bronchoconstriction.

Partial agonists: These have less intensity in their effect as a full agonist. However, they may prevent the action of other agonists and therefore may appear to be acting as antagonists. It is the mixture of actions which is called partial antagonism.

Interaction with enzymatic processes

Drugs can also work by interacting or interfering with enzymatic processes. Enzymes mediate many processes in the body, for example breakdown of alcohol and formation of cholesterol. They are catalytic proteins that increase the rate of chemical reactions in the body.

Inhibition of enzymes can lead to four effects:

- Cellular function – For example phosphodiesterone inhibitors (caffeine, theophylline) block the formation of a second messenger, which in the lungs can cause bronchodilation.
- Intermediary metabolism: For example allopurinol inhibits xanthine oxidase and thereby reduces the formation of uric acid from purines.
- Synthesis of mediators – For example prostaglandins formed by cyclooxygenase. Aspirin and other NSAIDs inhibit the

enzyme cyclooxygenase and therefore affect prostaglandin synthesis which is involved in inflammation.

- Degradation of chemical mediators – For example entacapone prevents the breakdown of levadopa; therefore, it has a much longer effect.

Interaction with transport systems

The lipid cell membrane provides a barrier against the transport of hydrophilic molecules into or out of a cell. For example, only lipid-soluble molecules can diffuse across a membrane. Ions and small water-soluble molecules, for example glucose and amino acids, can only cross membranes with the help of carrier proteins. Ion channels are selective pores in the membrane that allow the transfer of ions down their electrochemical gradient (concentration gradient). The open–closed state of these channels is controlled by either the membrane potential (voltage-sensitive channels) or transmitter substances.

Some channels, for example calcium channels in the heart, are both voltage and transmitter sensitive. Drugs that act on these channels include calcium antagonists (calcium channel blockers, e.g. nifedipine) and local anaesthetics. Anaesthetics block the channel physically and calcium antagonists bind to the channel protein, affecting the ability of drugs to interact across such channels and control heart rate and arrhythmias or vasodilation in the circulatory system.

Active transport processes are used to transfer substances against their concentration gradient. They use special carrier molecules in the membrane and require metabolic energy. These proteins have recognition sites for specific ions or molecules, which can be inhibited by drugs, for example digoxin, on the sodium/potassium pump and omeprazole on the proton pump. Two examples are as given as follows:

- The sodium pump expels sodium ions from the inside of the cell by a mechanism that derives energy from the enzyme ATPase. The carrier is linked to the transfer of potassium ions into the cell. The cardiac glycosides act by inhibiting the sodium/potassium-ATPase and compete with potassium for this. This is why patients are more sensitive to the effects of these drugs in the event of hypokalaemia. Sodium and chloride transport processes in the kidney are inhibited by some diuretics

• Noradrenaline transport into nerve terminals is responsible for inactivating the transmitter following its release into the synaptic cleft. The tricyclic antidepressants prolong the action of noradrenaline by blocking its reuptake

Drug licensing process – how are drugs licensed in the United Kingdom?

Many plants and other natural substances contain ingredients that have useful pharmacologic properties and actions. It is from the discovery of these and traditional methods of healing that modern pharmaceutical companies have developed the drugs that we have in the world now.

Until 1995, the only way to license a drug in the United Kingdom was through the Medicines Control Agency (MCA), now called the Medicines and Healthcare products Regulatory Agency (MHRA). But in 1995, the European Union established an organisation called the European Medicines Evaluation Agency (EMEA). Therefore, there are two ways a drug can be licensed for use in the United Kingdom, through either of these agencies.

After a product has been launched, doctors and other prescribers are allowed to prescribe it, either on the national health service (NHS) or through private health care, but only for people who meet the specific criteria of the drugs license. This often includes specific stages or types of a disease; for example a drug may be licensed for one type of cancer, but not another. In practice, some prescribers are not happy to prescribe a new drug at this early stage. There may be a lack of information available about side effects or long-term safety. These drugs are highlighted in the BNF by a black triangle.

For prescribing on the NHS, some hospitals and primary care trusts will not let their staff prescribe new drugs until they have been approved by National institute for health and care excellence

(NICE) (in England and Wales) and Scottish medicines consortium (SMC) (in Scotland). These organisations look at the evidence on how well the drug works, on any drawbacks or limitations and on cost-effectiveness. Ultimately, there is such a large amount of this work to do as it is so time consuming that there is often a backlog of new treatments waiting for approval.

Stages of drug development

The development of a new drug can take up to about ten years at times and cost millions of pounds. For every drug successfully developed, thousands are not and this is a cost to the pharmaceutical companies due to time and resources put into their development which is then not successful. The first stage in drug development is the research to find a new compound or combination of previously discovered and developed drugs. Following this pre-clinical trials are carried out, and these are usually in vitro or animal studies and involve pharmacological testing to discover much of the drug's potential effects and properties. All the results of these pre-clinical trials are evaluated, and then the clinical trials start where healthy volunteers are recruited. These are split into three phases. Phase 1 trials include a small number of subjects (healthy adults/subjects) and usually a relatively small number, for example 100. These trials will hopefully identify any obvious toxicity and safety problems. They focus on the clinical pharmacology of the drug and also the likely dosage of the end drug which will be required to have the therapeutic effects. Following the evaluation of the results from Phase 1 trials, Phase 2 trials are carried out and involve a greater number of subjects, for example about 500. These trials concentrate on piloting the efficacy and safety dose ranging. Phase 3 trials then include more subjects, for example about 3,000, and they examine major efficacy and safety dose ranging. These are full-scale clinical trials, and if the drug demonstrates safety and efficacy, then it will be marketed.

When the development of the drug reaches this stage, all the evidence gathered is then analysed and a report submitted for registration and licensing. The drug then goes through the marketing and product launch and is released into the marketplace for prescribers. Monitoring doesn't stop and post-marketing surveillance continues; this is sometimes referred to as Phase 4. The drug is identified as a black triangle drug as it is new, and the yellow card system of drug monitoring is in place (UKMI, 2003).

Drug interactions and polypharmacy

The term "polypharmacy" refers to the use of multiple medications by a patient. The most common outcomes of polypharmacy are increased adverse drug reactions and drug interactions and higher costs. Although polypharmacy is most abundant in the elderly, it is also widespread in the general population.

"Pill burden" is a term commonly used and refers to the number of tablets, capsules or other dosage forms that a patient takes on a regular basis. High pill burden decreases in compliance with drug therapy. It also increases the possibility of adverse medication reactions (side effects) and drug interactions. It has been associated with an increased risk of hospitalisation, medication errors and increased costs for both the drugs themselves and the treatment of the adverse events. It is also a source of dissatisfaction for many patients.

Polypharmacy is common in adults with chronic diseases, also having multiple conditions and being prescribed more than a dozen medications at times for all their respective conditions on a daily basis. The adverse reactions of these combinations of drugs are not reliably predictable. Because chronic conditions tend to accumulate in the elderly, polypharmacy is a particular issue here. There is also an added factor of alterations in drug pharmacokinetics and pharmacodynamics in the elderly (as discussed in Chapter 3).

Ways of reducing polypharmacy include selecting fixed-dose combination drug products, products with long-acting active ingredients and sustained release formulations when appropriate. Patients at greatest risk of polypharmacy are, as said previously, the elderly, but also psychiatric patients, patients taking five or more drugs concurrently, those with multiple doctors and health care professionals especially when they can all prescribe, individuals with multiple conditions, patients with low levels of education and those with impaired sight or dexterity.

Adverse drug reactions

An adverse effect is an unwanted effect of a drug. Adverse effects can be due to either toxic effects which arise through an exaggeration of the same pharmacological effect that is responsible for the effect of the drug, for example hypokalaemia, due to too high dose of diuretics, or side effects which are adverse effects that arise from a pharmacological action other than that which produces the therapeutic effect (the intended action). These may be dose related (e.g. symptoms heightened) or not (e.g. rash formation).

Adverse drug reactions (ADRs) may make a drug less effective, cause unexpected side effects or increase the action of a particular drug. Some ADRs can even cause physical and psychological harm to a person. ADRs fall into three broad categories;

1   Drug–drug interactions, which occur when two or more drugs react together with each other
2   Drug–food/beverage interactions, which result from drugs reacting with foods or beverages. For example, mixing alcohol with some drugs can alter the metabolism of that drug
3   Drug–condition interactions, which may occur when an existing medical condition makes certain drugs potentially harmful. For example, in renal disease sometimes a reduction in dose is required to avoid adverse reactions due to the decreased efficiency of drug excretion/elimination, which can result from a build-up of metabolites waiting to be excreted from the body

Over-the-counter (OTC) drugs can often have interactions with other drugs, and also some complementary therapies can have interactions with prescribed medications. For a full list of drug–drug interactions, see appendix 1 of the BNF. This should always be consulted before you start to prescribe multiple drugs.

Drug allergy/hypersensitivity reactions

Factors involved in drug allergy concern both the drug and the patient themselves. Some drugs have immunogenic components such as vaccines, enzymes such as streptokinase and polypeptides such as insulin. These can trigger immunological reactions. The patient themselves may have genetic factors which predispose them to be more prone to develop allergic drug reactions. They may have a history of allergic conditions such as asthma, eczema or hay fever or hereditary angio-oedema, which may make them more prone to allergic drug reactions.

Drug allergy and its manifestations should be classifiable according to the classification of the hypersensitivity reactions that occur. These are Type I–IV. However, in clinical practice, it is not always easy to fit a reaction into a specific classification.

Type I reactions/immediate hypersensitivity

These reactions involve interactions with immunoglobulin E (IgE) molecules which are attached to certain cells in the body (e.g. mast cells), for example anaphylaxis. The interaction triggers a set of cell reactions, which leads to the release of a number of chemical mediators such as histamine and kinins, which then cause the allergic response. The clinical manifestations of these reactions include urticarial, rhinitis, asthma symptoms, angio-oedema and even anaphylaxic shock. Drugs that most commonly cause these types of reactions include penicillin, local anaesthetics, streptomycin and radio opaque iodine which is sued as contract media in X-rays and scanning.

Type II reactions/cytotoxic reactions

These reactions involve the circulating antibodies of the immunoglobulin G, M or A (IgG, IgM or IgA) class, interacting with an antigen formed by a drug combined with a protein in a cell. Many of these reactions are haematological in nature, for example skin bruising and development of haematological anaemias and immune neutropenia.

Type III reactions/immune complex reactions

In these reactions, antibody (IgG) combines with antigen (e.g. a drug–protein complex) in the circulation. The complex formed is then deposited in the tissues, and complement is activated which then damages the endothelium of the capillaries. An example of this form of reaction is serum sickness, caused by penicillin, streptomycin, sulphonamides and antithyroid drugs. The symptoms that occur are fever, arthritis, enlarged lymph nodes, urticarial and maculopapular rashes.

Type IV reactions/cell-mediated or delayed hypersensitivity

In these reactions, T lymphocytes are sensitised by a drug–protein antigenic complex. When the lymphocytes come into contact with the antigen, an inflammatory response occurs. An example of this is contact dermatitis caused by anti-inflammatory creams or topical antibiotics.

Reporting ADRs/Yellow Card Scheme

Some side effects are not known about until many people have been taking the medicine for a while, thus the importance of reporting such events is important to raise awareness for future safety (BMA, 2006). It is especially useful to know about

1   A suspected side effect that is not mentioned on the drug information leaflet which is supplied with the medicine.
2   A suspected side effect that causes problems bad enough to interfere with everyday activities.
3   A suspected side effect that happens when taking two or more medicines and could be caused by interactions.

The Yellow Card Scheme is vital in helping the medicines and healthcare products regulatory agency (MHRA) monitor the safety of the medicines that are on the market. Yellow card reports (see the yellow card form at the back of the BNF) are evaluated together with additional sources of information such as clinical trial data, medical literature or data from international medicines regulators, in order to identify previously unidentified safety issues or side effects. Information gathered from the yellow card reports is continually assessed at the MHRA by a team of medicine safety experts, who study the benefits and risks of medicines. If a new side effect is identified, information is carefully considered in the context of the overall side effect profile for the medicine and how the side effect profile compares with other medicines used to treat the same condition. For more information on the yellow card scheme, see www.yellowcard.gov.uk, and for more information on the MHRA, see www.mhra.gov.uk.

The MHRA enters all the yellow card reports into a specialised database that allows rapid processing and analysis of all the information. This ongoing monitoring of drug safety is paramount for patient safety. Sometimes drugs will be withdrawn from the market if it is believed that risks are greater than the positive gains.

A monthly bulletin produced by the MHRA called "Drug Safety Update" gives health professionals updated information on the latest safety issues and guidance on the use of certain medicines. A free email service of this bulletin can be found at www.mhra.gov.uk/mhra/drugsafetyupdate.

Self-assessment test

1 What is the difference between the brand name and the generic name of a drug?
2 Give a simple definition of the term "pharmacodynamics".
3 What is a receptor?
4 Name the three types of receptors.
5 List the three ways drugs can act on the body.
6 List the four effects that can occur when enzymes are inhibited.
7 What are ion channels?

8 What is active transport?
9 What are the four processes involved in pharmacokinetics?
10 Name ten routes of administration of a drug.
11 What is the first–pass effect?
12 When does passive transfer occur and what determines its rate?
13 Name three factors that can affect the rate of absorption.
14 When does protein binding occur?
15 How many phases is the metabolism of drugs divided up into?
16 What family of enzymes is involved in Phase 1 reactions of drug metabolism?
17 When does conjugation occur and what is it?
18 Name the two important effects of drug metabolism.
19 What are the three mechanisms of excretion of drugs in the kidney?
20 What is meant by the term "bioavailability"?
21 What is a black triangle drug?
22 At what stage in the development of a drug is it trialled on actual people?
23 What are the most common outcomes of polypharmacy?
24 What does the term "pill burden" refer to?
25 Which groups of patients is polypharmacy more common in?
26 What are ADRs?
27 Which part of the BNF would you refer to, to look up about drug interactions?
28 What is the Yellow Card Scheme?

Reflective exercise

You have now read through and studied the contents of this chapter, and it is time for you to reflect on what you have learnt and how you are going to relate this to your prescribing practice. From what you have learnt, consider how this will influence what you prescribe? Will the information that you have learnt change any of the prescribing decisions that you thought you may have had previously, and if so, what, how and why?

References

BMA board of science. (2006). *Reporting of adverse drug reactions; a guide for healthcare professionals.* London: BMA.

UK Medicines Information (UKMi). (2003). *The licensing of medicines; an overview of the licensing process as it applies to medicinal products in the UK.* Liverpool: North West Medicines Information Centre.

3 Prescribing in co-morbidities and individual differences

Alison Pooler

Introduction

There are many considerations to make when prescribing a drug. These include the patient's age, current medication, current health status and past medical history. Prescribing is a complex professional role and knowledge of all these factors ensures safe and effective prescribing.

This chapter looks at the issues of prescribing for people with co-morbidities such as renal and liver disease. It considers the implications of prescribing for children and the elderly and for the pregnant woman.

Learning objectives

By the end of this chapter, students should be able to

- Understand and relate to the issues around prescribing for a person with renal disease/impairment.
- Understand and relate to the issues around prescribing for a person with liver/hepatic disease or dysfunction.
- Understand the issues surrounding prescribing for children.
- Understand the issues surrounding prescribing for the elderly.
- Understand the issues around prescribing for pregnant women and during breastfeeding.
- Relate the issues of polypharmacy to their own clinical practice area and understand practices that can be out in place to limit the effects of polypharmacy.

Prescribing in patients with renal impairment

Renal impairment may be the result of a variety of renal or systemic disease, such as diabetic nephropathy, hypertension, cardiovascular disease (CVD) or systemic lupus erythematous. Normal ageing results in a decline in renal function due to loss of nephrons. Elderly patients should therefore be assumed to have some degree of renal impairment, and this needs to be considered when prescribing. This is done through checking renal function prior to prescribing any drug that requires dose modification.

Reasons for problems with medication in renal failure include the following:

1   Failure to excrete a drug or its metabolites at the optimum speed
2   Many side effects are tolerated poorly by patients in renal failure and sensitivity to some drugs increases
3   Some drugs cease to be effective when renal function is reduced

Many of these problems can be avoided or reduced by reducing the dose or by using an alternate drug. Drugs that are renally excreted may need to have their doses reduced in patients with renal insufficiency or end-stage renal disease. For prescribing purposes, renal impairment is usually divided into three stages:

*   Mild: glomerular filtration rate (GFR) 20–50 ml/minute, serum creatinine approximately 150–300 μmol/l
*   Moderate: GFR 10–20 ml/minute, serum creatinine approximately 300–700 μmol/l
*   Severe: GFR less than 10 ml/minute, serum creatinine >700 μmol/l

Patients with GFR about 50 ml/minute do not usually require any dosage adjustment.

Nephrotoxic drugs should, if possible, be avoided in patients with renal disease because the consequences of nephrotoxicity are likely to be more serious when the renal reserve is already reduced.

The situation may change if a patient begins dialysis, since some drugs will be removed by the dialysis. Dialysis may lead to the loss of therapeutic effect of some drugs. Drugs to which particular attention must be given include many antibiotics, H2 blockers, digoxin, anticonvulsants and non-steroidal anti-inflammatory drugs.

For many drugs with only minor or no dose-related side effects, very precise modification of the dose regimen is unnecessary and a simple scheme for dose reduction is sufficient. For more toxic drugs with a small safety margin, dose regimens based on the GFR should be used. The total daily maintenance dose of a drug can be reduced either by reducing the size of the individual doses or by increasing the interval between the doses. For some drugs, if the size of the maintenance dose is reduced, it will be important to give a loading dose if an immediate effect is required. The loading dose should usually be the same size as the initial dose for a patient with normal renal function (NICE, 2008).

Some drugs cause biochemical changes which can be dangerous, and these include the following:

- Prescribing any drug that increases potassium levels, which is potentially very dangerous, for example potassium supplements, potassium sparing diuretics and other products that contain potassium such as ispaghula husk laxatives.
- Products with high sodium content, e.g. some antacids, which may cause sodium and water retention in patients with renal impairment.
- Excessive vitamin D replacement therapy which can cause hypercalcaemia that may precipitate or exacerbate renal impairment. Many patients with chronic renal failure are prescribed alfacalcidol, and therapy should be monitored closely.

Nephrotoxic drugs

These drugs are classified as drugs that cause pre-renal damage, intra-renal damage, post-renal damage (urinary tract damage) and other nephrotoxic drugs.

Drugs causing pre-renal damage include drugs that cause gastrointestinal losses, through either diarrhoea or vomiting, and also volume depletion and may precipitate acute renal failure. Non-steroidal anti-inflammatory drugs (NSAIDs), even in short courses, can cause acute renal failure as a result of renal under perfusion. Angiotension-converting enzyme (ACE) inhibitors can also cause a deterioration in renal function. However, this is a problem only in patients with compromised renal perfusion, particularly those with renal artery stenosis. Care should be taken when an ACE inhibitor and NSAID are prescribed together as this combination may precipitate an acute deterioration in renal function.

Drugs causing intra-renal damage may result in direct damage on the kidneys or hypersensitivity reactions. Most drugs that cause damage within the kidney do so as a result of hypersensitivity reactions, which involve either glomerular or interstitial damage. Drugs that have been reported to cause glomerulonephritis include penicillamine, gold, captopril, phenytoin and some antibiotics, including penicillin, sulphonamides, thiazide diuretics, furosemide, NSAIDs and rifampicin. There are also a number of drugs that cause direct toxicity to the renal tubules (acute tubular necrosis), for example aminoglycosides, amphotericin and cyclosporine.

Drugs causing post-renal damage (urinary tract obstruction) include high-dose sulphonamides, acetazolamide or methotrexate, which may also cause crystalluria and could therefore cause obstruction. Anticholinergics (e.g. tricyclic antidepressants and alcohol) may cause urinary tract obstruction due to retention of urine in the bladder.

Other nephrotoxic drugs include cephalosporins (i.e. Cephaloridine, one of the first cephalosporins introduced) has been associated with direct renal toxicity and is no longer in clinical use. Other cephalosporins are much less likely to produce renal damage but third-generation cephalosporins (e.g. cefixime) have very rarely been reported to cause nephrotoxicity.

Another class of nephrotoxic drugs are analgesics, such as NSAIDs, which may cause acute renal failure due to hypo-perfusion and interstitial nephritis, as well as analgesic nephropathy (chronic interstitial nephritis and papillary necrosis). Analgesic nephropathy has been most commonly seen with combination analgesia products that contain aspirin and/or paracetamol. Analgesic nephropathy is one of the few preventable causes of chronic renal failure. Discontinuation of the abused drug often results in stabilisation or even improvement in renal function, but continued abuse leads to further renal damage.

Lithium is another nephrotoxic drug, and serum levels of lithium consistently above the therapeutic range have been associated with development of nephrogenic diabetes insipidus.

Effects on drug absorption from renal impairment

Renal impairment can affect the absorption of drugs by the following:

- Altered gastrointestinal motility and reduction in absorption caused through nausea, vomiting and diarrhoea
- Increased gastric ammonia that increases gastric pH and acidity which can affect the absorption of some drugs (e.g. digoxin and ferrous sulphate)
- Phosphate binders and calcium resonate which are used in the treatment of renal failure and can impede the absorption profile of slow release and enteric coated drugs

Effects on drug distribution from renal impairment

Renal impairment alters the volume of distribution due to fluid overload, reduced albumin and altered protein binding. The state of hydration of the patient will affect the volume of distribution for water-soluble drugs, and reduced protein binding due to uraemia changing the shape of binding sites affects drugs which have a high affinity to bind to plasma proteins. All the above affect the distribution of drugs around the body.

Effects on drug metabolism from renal impairment

Only a small number of drugs are metabolised in the kidneys. However, the kidneys are important in the role of degradation of insulin and the conversation of vitamin D to its active form. Therefore, some patients may need to have smaller doses of insulin if they have renal impairment.

Effects on drug elimination from renal impairment

As the kidneys are the main organs involved in drug elimination from the body, there can be considerable effects on this process if there is a degree of renal impairment. Water-soluble drugs and their water-soluble metabolites that are mainly excreted by the kidneys may have a prolonged half-life in renal impairment and can therefore accumulate and cause toxicity. Therefore, consideration may need to be given to lower the doses of some drugs or increase the dosage schedule to give more time between doses.

General principles of prescribing in renal disease

When prescribing in anyone who has any form of renal impairment or disease, the following principles need to be considered:

* Determine the presence and severity of renal impairment, using estimated glomerular filtration rate (eGFR) levels.
* Consider the psychological and social impact of the condition and its treatments, as they may have an impact on concordance with medications being taken by the patient.
* Only use a drug if there is an indication.
* Avoid nephrotoxic drugs and the information is found listed in the contraindications section of the British national formulary (BNF) for each drug.
* Use recommended dosage regimens from renal failure as detailed in the BNF under each drug entry.
* Review and monitor regularly.
* Refer to a real specialist if in any doubt.

Prescribing in patients with liver dysfunction

The metabolism of many drugs depends on adequate hepatic (liver) function. Drugs with a narrow therapeutic range (i.e. with little difference between toxic and therapeutic doses) run the risk of accumulating and causing toxicity in patients with liver disease.

The liver receives a dual blood supply with about 20% of the blood coming from the hepatic artery and 80% coming from the portal circulation. The blood flow to the liver is around 20–25% of the total cardiac output. Toxins, infectious agents, medications and serum inflammatory mediators may result in a diverse range of disease processes leading to loss of normal histological architecture, reduced cell mass and loss of blood flow. Consequently, functional liver capacity may be lost.

Assessing hepatic (liver) function is therefore necessary so that appropriate adjustment of drug dose can be made. However, this is not always straightforward as there is no single test that reliably measures liver function.

Drug metabolism in the liver

The liver is the principal organ of drug metabolism in the body, although other sites such as the gut wall, kidney, skin and lungs are involved. Drug metabolism, by means of enzyme reactions in the liver, is the body's main method of deactivating drugs. Drug molecules are converted into more polar compounds, which aid their elimination. Generally, metabolism results in the loss of pharmacological activity because transport to the site of action is limited due to reduced lipid solubility or because the molecule is no longer able to attach itself onto the receptor site. However, in some circumstances, drugs are metabolised to more active forms, for example the conversion of codeine to morphine, primidone to phenobarbitone and amitriptyline to nortriptyline.

Concentrations of enzymes involved in both phase I and phase II reactions vary significantly between individuals with normal hepatic function and even more so between the healthy population and those with hepatic impairment.

Phase I reactions

Most drugs are lipophilic and therefore readily cross the cell membrane of the enterocyte. In the process of liver metabolism, these substances are converted into more hydrophilic compounds. Hydrolysis, oxidation and reduction are the three types of phase I reactions that do this in the liver. These mainly involve a subset of monooxygenase enzymes called cytochrome P450 system. The most common reaction is hydrolysis which involves the addition of a molecular oxygen atom to form a hydroxyl group, with the other oxygen atom being converted to water, for example the conversion of aspirin to salicylic acid.

Other types of phase I reactions include oxidation via soluble enzymes such as alcohol dehydrogenase and reduction (e.g. nitrazepam).

Phase II reactions

These reactions involve conjugation which is the attachment of molecules naturally present in the body to a suitable link in the drug molecule. Most compounds will have undergone a phase I reaction (e.g. addition of a hydroxyl group) before the conjugation step can occur. The main conjugation reaction involves glucuronidation (e.g. morphine), but other conjugation mechanisms include acetylation (sulfonamides) or the addition of glycine (nicotinic acid) and sulphate (morphine). Natural substances such as bilirubin and thyroxine may be metabolised by the same pathways. The resulting conjugate molecule is usually pharmacologically inactive and substantially less lipophilic than its precursor so it is more readily excreted in the bile and urine.

In some circumstances, the parent compound is a prodrug so the metabolite is active; for example codeine is converted to morphine. A common cause of capacity-limited hepatic metabolism is the amount of the conjugate available. Paracetamol overdose is an example of this. With normal doses of paracetamol, the toxic metabolite is efficiently detoxified by conjugation with glutathione as a phase II reaction. However, when a large amount of the metabolite is generated, the total quantity of available glutathione may be consumed and the detoxifying process becomes overwhelmed. Phenytoin and warfarin are other drugs where capacity-limited hepatic metabolism can occur.

Excretion

Following metabolism, compounds are then either excreted directly into the bile or re-enter the systemic circulation and are excreted as polar metabolites or conjugates by the kidneys. If excreted in the bile (mainly glucuronidated drugs), the compound enters the biliary duct system and is secreted into the upper small intestine. Then throughout the ileum, these conjugated bile salts (some of which have drugs attached to them) are reabsorbed and transported back to the liver via the portal circulation. This is known as enterohepatic circulation.

Each bile salt is reused approximately 20 times and often repeatedly in the same digestive phase. The implications of this process are that compounds may reach high hepatic concentrations resulting in significant hepatotoxicity. Some drugs that undergo enterohepatic cycling to a significant extent include phenytoin, leflunomide and tetracycline antibiotics.

After drugs are absorbed from the gut, a proportion of the dose may be eliminated by the liver before reaching the systemic circulation. This pre-systemic or first-pass elimination is determined by the hepatic clearance or extraction for the compound. Hepatic clearance depends on three factors:

- Extent of drug binding to blood components such as albumin
- Blood flow to active metabolic cells, which is dependent on the architecture of the liver
- Functional hepatocytes

The hepatic extraction rate of a drug will indicate if its elimination is dependent on blood flow and hepatocyte function (highly extracted) or hepatocyte function alone (poorly extracted). Some examples of high extraction drugs are antidepressants, haloperidol, calcium channel blockers, morphine, levodopa and propanolol. Examples of low extraction drugs are NSAIDs, diazepam, carbamazepine, phenytoin and warfarin.

Hepatic conditions

Chronic liver disease is more predictably associated with impaired metabolism of drugs than acute liver dysfunction. However, in cases of severe acute liver failure, the capacity to metabolise the drug may be significantly impaired. In the chronic state, cirrhosis of any aetiology, viral hepatitis and hepatoma can decrease drug metabolism. In moderate to severe liver dysfunction, rates of drug metabolism may be reduced by as much as 50%. The mechanism is thought to be due to spatial separation of blood from the hepatocyte by fibrosis along the hepatic sinusoids.

The use of certain drugs in patients with cirrhosis occasionally increases the risk of hepatic decompensation. An example of this is the increased risk of hepatic encephalopathy in some patients who receive pegylated interferon alfa-2a in combination with ribavirin for the treatment of chronic active hepatitis, related to the hepatitis C virus.

In the presence of chronic liver disease, there is potential for changing the systemic availability of high extraction drugs, thereby affecting plasma concentrations. A potential consequence of liver disease is the development of portosystemic shunts that may carry a drug absorbed from the gut through the mesenteric veins directly into the systemic circulation. As such, oral treatment with high hepatic clearance drugs such as morphine or propanalol can lead to high plasma concentrations and an increased risk of adverse effects. Liver damage can also affect drugs with low hepatic clearance. For example, the effect on warfarin, which has a low extraction ratio, is increased due to the reduced production of vitamin K-dependent clotting factors.

The pharmacokinetic interaction between drugs and alcohol is more complex. An acute ingestion of alcohol may inhibit a drug's metabolism by competing with the drug for the same set of metabolising enzymes. Conversely, hepatic enzyme induction may occur with chronic excessive alcohol ingestion, resulting in increased clearance of certain drugs (e.g. phenytoin and benzodiazepines). After these enzymes have been induced, they remain so in the absence of alcohol for several weeks after cessation of drinking. In addition, some enzymes induced by chronic alcohol consumption transform some drugs (e.g. paracetamol) into toxic compounds that can cause further liver damage.

In the presence of cholestatic jaundice, drugs and their active metabolites that are dependent on biliary excretion for clearance will have impaired elimination. Further impairment will occur if the compound is excreted as a glucuronide and is subject to enterohepatic circulation.

Evaluating hepatic function

A clear patient history with respect to alcohol consumption, illicit drug use and toxic industrial exposure must be recorded. The medication list including supplements such as iron, vitamin A and herbal remedies is vital. A family history of diseases such as alpha-1 antitrypsin deficiency, iron storage diseases, porphyrias and diabetes mellitus may alert the health professional to the potential for liver impairment.

It is also important to look for signs of acute or chronic liver disease such as presence of jaundice, spider naevi, palmer erythema, ascites, abdominal distension, hepatomegaly and splenomegaly. If there is clinical evidence of liver disease, further investigation is required, which includes liver function tests and ultrasound of the abdomen. A portal vein Doppler may be recommended for assessing the presence of portal hypertension, which may be related to cirrhosis or portal vein thrombosis if the flow is reduced.

In renal disease, serum creatinine concentration and the GFR provide a reasonable guide to drug dosage requirements. In contrast, there is no single test that measures liver function so a reliable prediction of pharmacokinetics is not possible. Some evaluation of liver function is possible by assessing serum albumin and bilirubin and prothrombin time. However, these parameters are not directly related to drug clearance. Although not directly correlated with liver dysfunction, elevated liver enzymes may raise the suspicion of hepatic impairment requiring further investigation.

Evaluating the drug to be prescribed

If a drug is dependent on hepatic elimination, there are several factors to consider when prescribing for patient with liver disease.

- Ascertain how much the drug depends on hepatic metabolism for its elimination from the body.
- If there is any doubt about the degree of hepatic impairment or the drug has a narrow therapeutic index, then lower the recommended starting dose by approximately 50% and titrate to effect under supervision (start low and go slow).
- Determine possible interactions between the new drug and any drugs that are already prescribed.

Determining the hepatic contribution to elimination is paramount and the following general rules should be considered:

1   Drugs with a narrow therapeutic range that are extensively metabolised by the liver (>20% of their metabolism) should either be avoided altogether (e.g. pethadine) or used with extreme caution (e.g. morphine and theophylline) in patients with significant liver disease.

2   Drugs with a wide therapeutic range which also undergo extensive hepatic metabolism should be used with caution. In particular, the dosing interval should be increased or the total dose reduced (e.g. carvedilol).

3   If hepatic elimination is limited, then the therapeutic range of the compound should be reviewed. If the drug has a wide therapeutic index, then the likelihood of an adverse effect related to hepatic impairment is low. However, if the drug has a narrow therapeutic index, then caution should be exercised and significant hepatic impairment may have a clinically relevant effect on the pharmacokinetics.

Prescribing in hepatic impairment is less well defined when compared to guidelines for prescribing in renal failure. Hepatic dysfunction is less overt and may not be apparent until much of the functioning liver is lost. Knowledge of the metabolism of drugs eliminated by the liver is useful along with close monitoring of the patient for unwanted side effects related to possible toxicity. When introducing long-term treatment with a drug with high hepatic clearance or a narrow therapeutic range, assess liver function (clinically and with liver function blood tests). However, once a drug is commenced, routine monitoring is costly and its role is unclear in most cases of prescribing in patient with hepatic dysfunction.

Prescribing for children

Children and particularly neonates differ from adults in their response to drugs. Special care is needed in ensuring that the drug prescribed is appropriate and that the correct dosage is given, especially in the neonatal period.

Factors affecting pharmacokinetic processes of drugs in children

Absorption of drugs administered orally

1   Variable gastric and intestinal transit time: In young infants, gastric emptying time is prolonged and only approaches adult values at around six months of age. In older infants, intestinal hurry may occur.
2   Increased gastric pH: Gastric acid output does not reach adult values until the second year of life.
3   Other factors: Gastrointestinal contents, posture, disease states and therapeutic interventions such as drug therapy can also affect the absorption process.

Distribution of drugs

1   Increased total body water: As a percentage of total body weight, the total body water and extracellular fluid volume decrease with increasing age. Neonates require higher doses of water-soluble drugs on an mg/kg basis than adults.
2   Decreased plasma protein binding: Plasma protein binding in neonates is reduced as a result of low levels of albumin and globulins and an altered binding capacity. High circulating bilirubin levels in neonates may displace drugs from albumin.

Metabolism of drugs

1   Enzyme systems mature at different times and may be absent at birth or present in considerably reduced amounts.
2   Altered metabolic pathways may exist for some drugs.
3   Metabolic rate increases dramatically in children and is often greater than in adults. Compared with adults, children may require more frequent dosing or higher doses on an mg/kg basis.

Excretion of drugs

Complete maturation of renal function is not reached until six to eight months of age.

Route of administration and drug regimes

Compliance in children is influenced by the formulation, taste, appearance and ease of administration of a preparation. Prescribed regimens should therefore be tailored to the child's daily routine, and, where possible, treatment goals should be set in collaboration with the child and/or family.

Wherever possible, the use of products which avoid the need for administration during school hours should be considered due to the restrictions now in play within the education authority. For example, consider slow release medications which have a long half-life and the need to administer twice a day rather than four times a day. When administration during school time is unavoidable, consideration should be given to prescribing and supplying the school time dose in a separate labelled container. Most schools will request written permission and instructions on how to administer the drugs, and others will ask the parents to come to school to administer the drug themselves to their child.

Wherever possible, painful intramuscular (IM) injections should be avoided and the use of props and companions such as teddy bears should be considered for the younger children, and demonstration using the toy to teach the child that takes the drug is OK to do.

Product licence for children

Wherever possible, medicines should be prescribed within the terms of the product licence. However, many children may require medicines not specifically licensed for paediatric use. The Medicines Act 1968 and European legislation make provision for prescribers to use medicines in an off-label capacity or to use unlicensed medicines. However, individual prescribers are always responsible for ensuring that there is adequate information to support he quality, efficacy, safety and intended use of a drug before prescribing it.

Although medicines cannot be promoted outside the limits of the licence, the Medicine Act does not prohibit the use of unlicensed medicines. It is recognised that the informed use of unlicensed medicines or of licence drugs for unlicensed application (off label use) is often necessary in paediatric practice. Hence, accurate record keeping must be ensured by the prescriber in any off-licence prescribing.

Prescription writing for children

There are a number of principles to bear in mind when writing a prescription for a child, and these are as follows:

- Inclusion of age is a legal requirement in the case of prescription only medicines for children under 12 years of age, but it is preferable to state the age for all prescriptions for children. It is particularly important to state the strengths of capsules or tablets.
- Although liquid preparations are particularly suitable for children, they may contain sugar which encourages dental decay. Sugar-free medicines are preferred for long-term treatment. Many children are able to swallow tablets or capsules and may prefer a solid dose form, involving the child and parents in choosing the formulation is helpful in compliance
- When a prescription for a liquid oral preparation is written and the dose ordered is smaller than 5 ml, an oral syringe will be supplied.
- Parents should be advised not to add any medicines to infants feeds, since the drug may interact with the milk or other liquid in it; moreover, the ingested dosage may be reduced if the child does not drink all the contents.

Dosages for children

Children are not mini adults. Paediatric doses should be obtained from the paediatric dose reference text and not extrapolated from the adult dose. When considering drug use in children, the following age groups should be referred to

- Neonate (birth to one month)
- Infant (one month to two years)

- Child (2–12 years)
- Adolescent (12–18 years)

Unless the age is specified, the term "child" in the BNF includes persons aged 12 years and under.

Child doses may be calculated from the adult doses by using age, body weight or body surface area, or by a combination of these factors. The most reliable methods rely on body surface area. Body weight may be used to calculate doses expressed in mg/kg. Younger children may require a higher dose per kilogram being administered. In such cases, dose should be calculated on the ideal weight related to height and age (there is a simple table at the back of the BNF for this).

Body surface area estimates are more accurate for calculation of paediatric doses than body weight, since many physiological phenomena correlate better to body surface area. BSA may be calculated from height and weight by means of a monogram or using the body surface area (BSA) calculator which is found in the BNF.

Adverse drug reactions that can occur in children

Adverse drug reaction (ADR) profiles may differ from those seen in adults. All prescribers should report any suspected ADR to the Medicines and Healthcare products Regulatory Agency (MHRA), even if the product is being used in an off-label manner or is an unlicensed product. The identification and reporting of adverse reactions to drugs in children is particularly important because

- The action of the drug and its pharmacokinetics in children (especially in the very young) may differ from that in adults.
- Drugs are not extensively tested in children.
- Many drugs are not specifically licensed for use in children and are used off-label.
- Suitable formulations may not be available to allow precise dosing in children.
- The nature and course of illnesses and ADRs may differ between adults and children.

Prescribing in the elderly

The elderly are major consumers of drugs, and most prescribers of whatever speciality will regularly prescribe for the elderly. The principles of geriatric pharmacology are well established, and most prescribers will automatically modify their prescribing habits when dealing with elderly patients (Reddy, 2006).

Excessive prescribing is common in the elderly. The over 65s comprise between 12% and 18% of developed populations; despite this, they receive up to 40% of all prescriptions. Furthermore, there is a progressive and age-related rise in drug usage, most marked in females. Detailed analysis of drug utilisation in the elderly suggests that almost two-thirds may be taking either prescribed or over-the-counter medications at any one time. This is partly because most common chronic diseases become more prevalence in the elderly, but the widespread use of drugs such as diuretics, agnates active on the nervous system and NSAIDs suggests that excess prescribing is a continuing problem (Kings Fund, 2013).

Treatment alternatives and quality of life

Many common problems of the elderly do not necessarily require pharmacological intervention, and many health care professional use other therapeutic approaches as an initial stage of treatment. For example, insomnia is a common problem in the elderly, and it may be more appropriate to prescribe a hot milky drink and a good book rather than sleeping tablets. Physiotherapy can be used in arthritis and can be more successful than the use of NSAIDs and less risky in terms of long-term side effects.

Compliance and information

It was thought that compliance with medication in the elderly was worse than adults, but this was found not to be true. Compliance only seems to be an issue where there is cognitive impairment. For those with mild problems, memory joggers such as drug diaries and pre-loaded drug boxes may be helpful. For the markedly demented, there is no alternative other than supervised drug administration by formal or informal carers. Drug information leaflets, counselling by pharmacists, nurse and doctors and training as part of rehabilitation programme all improve compliance and should be part of the routine geriatric multidisciplinary package.

It should also be considered that many elderly arthritic patients may find it difficult to open packaging and containers. A variety of special tablet bottles are now available. Many elderly also have poor eyesight and find it difficult to read the prescribing information, so provision of large print could be used.

Lower starting dose

When prescribing for the elderly, a lower starting dose is used. The reason for this is simple: the elderly are more sensitive to a given dose of a drug. For example, the starting dose of nifedipine is 20 mg in an adult but 10 mg in the elderly. There are many reasons for this increased sensitivity, relating to pharmacokinetics and pharmacodynamics and also loss of homeostatic reserve.

Pharmacokinetic changes in the elderly

Bioavailability of a drug is markedly influenced by changes in hepatic pre-systemic (first-pass) metabolism. When a drug is taken orally, the medicine disperses in the stomach, passes to the small bowel and is absorbed. It enters the portal system and is carried to the liver. For some compounds, hepatic extraction is relatively low and most of the absorbed doses will transverse the liver without significant uptake. For these agents, age-related changes in the first-pass hepatic metabolism are probably limited significance. However, some compounds are avidly taken up by the liver on this first pass through it (sometimes well over 90–95% of the drug is removed). This results in a very significantly reduced bioavailability. A reduction in first-pass metabolism from 95% to 90% in an elderly person would result in an increase in bioavailability from 5% to 10%, which is doubled. This is why reduced dosage requirements are necessary in highly extracted drugs.

Pharmacodynamic changes in the elderly

Changes in receptor function are modified as part of the normal ageing process. The changes are complex and not always in the same direction. For example, elderly people seem to be paradoxically resistant to agents acting on beta receptors, possibly because of loss of high-affinity receptor subtypes. By contrast, old people are particularly sensitive to warfarin, require a lower maintenance dose and may be very sensitive to coumarin anticoagulants.

Changes in central nervous system receptors occur which may lead the elderly person to be more susceptible to confusion and the sedative effects of psychoactive drugs. Changes in dopamine receptor subtypes lead elderly individuals to be particularly prone to develop extra pyramidal side effects when exposed to dopamine blockers.

Homeostatic failure

A feature of the ageing process is loss of adaptability. This is most obviously manifested with regard to postural blood pressure control. In young individuals, assuming the upright posture is associated by a transient fall in blood pressure, this is noted by baroreceptors in the carotid sinus and elsewhere, resulting in reflex tachycardia and subsequent peripheral vascular vasoconstriction. In the elderly, this set of reflexes is blunted or lost, reflex tachycardia is less marked and vasoconstriction may be slower. This leads the elderly to be particularly at risk from postural hypotension when given vasodilating agents and may result in falls.

Postural control may be regarded as a homeostatic mechanism and may easily be measured by determination of body sway. Body say is greater in drug-free normal elderly than in the young; this is considerably magnified when they are exposed to drugs acting on the central nervous system and may once more be another cause of falls.

Thermoregulation is a basic homeostatic response. Although thermoregulatory responses are not blunted in all elderly people, they are certainly impaired in survivors of accidental hypothermia and such individuals are more frequent in the elderly age groups.

Extended dosing interval

In addition to choosing lower starting dose, prescribers frequently extend the dosing interval when prescribing for the elderly. Drugs may, for example, be given twice a day instead of thrice a day. The reason for this is that many agents have a slower elimination in the elderly compared to the young.

The two prime sites of drug elimination are the liver and kidney, and considerable information is now available on the relationship between ageing and the physiology of these agents.

Hepatic drug elimination

Elimination of drugs by the liver is reduced in the elderly. This relates to the morphological and physiological changes in the liver, that is the liver is smaller and with a lower blood flow. Ultrasound has shown that there is a decline in liver mass, even allowing for changes in body weight, of approximately 35% between the ages of 29 and 90. A similar perhaps slightly greater fall in liver blood flow also occurs. These changes in hepatic morphology are easily of sufficient magnitude to explain impaired hepatic drug elimination in the elderly.

Renal drug elimination

Most aspects of renal function fall in the elderly, although the degree of impairment varies considerably between individuals. GFR, effective renal plasma flow and renal tubular function are all reduced in the elderly. For example, the GFR of a 20-year-old may be 120 ml/min, and that of a 90-year-old 30 ml/min. Clearly drugs that are eliminated by the kidney will have significantly delayed elimination in the elderly, leading to higher plasma concentrations and the development of toxicity.

Particularly important agents so affected include aminogly-coside antibiotics such as gentamycin and streptomycin, some beta-blockers and lithium. An extension of dosing interval will overcome these problems.

Treatment review and monitoring for adverse reactions

It is often forgotten that drug treatment even for relatively chronic illnesses may not be continually required. For example, severity of arthritic pain varies considerably with time; many patients who have been given diuretics for ankle swelling and mild congestive cardiac failure may not require these drugs on an indefinite basis. Regular review of treatment is therefore mandatory and should be facilitated in primary care by computerised records and prescription information.

Monitoring for adverse reactions is fundamental. You may assume that if all the above guidelines are assiduously followed, then adverse reactions in the elderly would be infrequent. This is not the case. Adverse reactions are most prevalent in the elderly population, particularly elderly women. Eighty per cent of these reactions are type A dose dependent and are simply due to the patient being exposed to too high a dose of the drug at too frequent a dosing interval for them. This poses a public health issue as up to 25% of acute admission of the elderly is due to ADRs.

Summary of principles to consider when prescribing in the elderly

When prescribing any medications in elderly patients, the following principles need to be considered;

- Ensure effective communication with the elderly person and their family if necessary.
- Keep drug regimens simple.
- Consider reminder charts, doset boxes, concordance aids and written instructions.
- Monitor concordance by counting the number of tablets taken or by monitoring plasm levels of drugs if necessary.

- Review medications regularly and monitor repeat prescriptions.
- Stop any medication which is not required.
- Consider potential practical difficulties such as opening bottle or small containers.
- Consider poor vision and swallowing difficulties when prescribing drugs and how instructions are given to the patient.

Prescribing in pregnancy

The potential for doing harm to the foetus by prescribing drugs for the mother during pregnancy is considerable, as was seen with the thalidomide disaster. About 35% of women take drug therapy at least once during pregnancy and 6% during the first trimester (this excludes iron, folic acid and vitamins). The most commonly used drugs are simple analgesics, antibacterial drugs and antacids. However, drugs should only be given to pregnant women if the likely benefit to the mother outweighs the risk to the foetus. In general, only those drugs should be prescribed of which there is extensive experience in human pregnancy. This is usually not the case with newly introduced drugs. In rare cases, a drug is given to the mother for a specific therapeutic effect on the foetus.

Altered pharmacokinetics in pregnancy

Absorption: The extent of absorption of drugs is generally unaltered in pregnancy, although the rate of absorption may be reduced because of a reduced rate of gastric emptying. Vomiting is common in pregnancy and can affect drug administration.

Distribution: Plasma volume increases by about 50% and total body water by about 20% during late pregnancy. Thus, if the apparent volume of distribution of a drug is usually low, it will increase significantly. However, this is generally not of great clinical importance, firstly because steady-state plasma concentrations are independent of the apparent volume of distribution and secondly because although an increase in volume causes an increase in the half-life, this is usually more than offset by an increase in clearance, due to reduced protein binding and increased metabolism.

Plasma albumin concentrations fall by up to 10 g/l during pregnancy. There can therefore be a fall in the bound fraction of drugs that normally are bound extensively to plasma albumin. For example, there is an increase in the unbound fraction of phenytoin in the plasma during pregnancy and as a result total plasma phenytoin concentrations fall because of increased clearance. However, the concentration of unbound phenytoin does not fall to the same extent, and great care must be taken in adjusting dosages and in interpreting plasma concentration measurements.

Metabolism: Because of the ethical problems of carrying out drug studies in pregnant women, there is not much information about drug metabolised in pregnancy. Indirect evidence such as liver histology and urine excretion suggests that drug metabolism is increased in pregnancy, and this is consistent with the observed increase in the clearance rate of theophyline in pregnancy. In contrast, there is no increase in blood flow to the liver during pregnancy, and the clearance of drugs whose hepatic excretion ratio is high does not change.

Excretion: in pregnancy the GFR increases by about 70%. Thus drugs that are eliminated mainly by renal excretion are cleared more quickly. The dosage requirements of lithium and digoxin therefore increase during pregnancy and plasma concentrations monitoring will help to guide therapy, as dosages may need to be increased.

Tetragenesis

This is the occurrence of a developmental abnormality in a foetus in response to the effect of a drug taken during the early stages of pregnancy. Reliable information is hard to find about this in humans and animal studies don't always relate to humans. For a drug to affect the development of a foetus, tt must first pass across the placental barrier. The mechanisms whereby drugs pass across the placenta are similar to those that pass across any lipid membrane and most drugs pass across by simple diffusion.

The first trimester of pregnancy and particularly the periods between weeks 2 and 8 is most crucial as this is when the organs are starting to develop (organogenesis). During this time, drugs can cause structural abnormalities. Later in foetal life, drugs can affect the subsequent growth, development and integrity of the body structures, particularly the brain. Any drug that is taken by a non-pregnant woman but that is stored and released later during the time that she conceives is also potentially dangerous. An example of this is the retinoid etretinate, a definite tetrogenic drug that is used in the treatment of severe acne and psoriasis, accumulates in the subcutaneous fat, from which it is released very slowly. Women who take this drug should be advised to stop the drug two months prior to trying to get pregnant. If a drug is known to be a tetrogenon in human or animals, then it is stated on the data sheet. However, if this is not known, then only advice can be given to use with caution, especially during the first trimester.

Table 3.1 lists some drugs that should be avoided during pregnancy and the reasons why. This only shows some of the drugs, and the current BNF should be consulted for the full up-to-date

Table 3.1 Drugs that should be avoided during early pregnancy (due to high risk of causing abortion)

Drug	Effect
Alcohol	Foetal alcohol syndrome
Androgens	Multiple congenital abnormalities
Antineoplastic agents (e.g. methotrexate)	Multiple congenital defects
Carbimazole	Aplasia cutis
Corticosteroids (high doses)	Cleft palate
Cyproterone	Feminisation of male foetus
Diethylstilbesterol	Vaginal adenosis and adenocarcinoma in daughters
Distigmine	Increases uterine tone
Ergotamine	Increases uterine tone
Misoprostol	Increases uterine tone
Fibrinolytic drugs (e.g. streptokinase)	Placental separation
Tetracyclines	Yellow discolourisation of teeth and inhibition on bone growth
Valporate	Neural tubal defects
vitamin A	Congenital defects
Warfarin	Multiple congenital defects

Source: BNF (2020).

list. Information can also be found at the National Teratology Information Service (NTIS) regional drug and therapeutics centre www.uktris.org. If there is any doubt, then do not prescribe.

Adverse effects of drugs on the foetus during the later stages of pregnancy

Some drugs are not tetrogenic but can have adverse effects on the foetus if given later in pregnancy. These include drugs that can be given immediately before labour and can cause problems in the neonate.

Aspirin: It has been suggested to be tetragenic in early pregnancy, but the case has not been proven. However, in high doses in late pregnancy, it can displace foetal bilirubin from plasma proteins and thus cause kernicterus. Also if taken within one week of delivery, it can cause impaired haemostasis in the mother during labour and haemorrhage in the neonate. Low–dose aspirin has been used as an antiplatelet agent in the hope of preventing pre-eclampsia. Although results are not encouraging, there seem to be no ill effects to the foetus, but there is a slight risk of increased bleeding in the mother at the time of delivery

Aminoglycoside antibiotics: These should be used only if really necessary due the effects on the eight nerve.

Antithyroid drugs: These can be used during pregnancy but at the minimum dose necessary to control maternal hypothyroidism. Some recommend using half the normal dose.

Benzodiazipines: If given at the time around labour, they can cause the floppy infant syndrome, with muscular hypotonia, hypothermia, respiratory difficulties and difficulty with sucking.

Choramphenicol: It is poorly metabolised by the immature liver and can cause peripheral vascular collapse if given to neonates in weight-corrected adult doses. It should not be used at all during pregnancy.

Oral anticoagulants: These are tetrogenic during the first trimester and can also cause foetal or retroplacental haemorrhage if given late in pregnancy. They should be avoided at all costs in early and late stages of pregnancy. Some people avoid warfarin completely and rely on subcutaneous heparin instead. Heparin does not cross the placenta and is therefore relatively safe.

Pethidine: Care should be taken not to give too much due to respiratory depression in the neonate. Babies who are born to mothers who have an addiction to narcotic analgesics have a narcotic withdrawal syndrome after delivery, especially if they are given naloxone.

Tetracyclines: These should not be used at any time because of their effects on growing teeth and bones.

Thiazide diuretics: These can cause thrombocytopenia in the neonate, probably by a direct toxic effect on the marrow and should be avoided in late pregnancy.

Drug therapy and breastfeeding

The problem of adverse effects in suckling infants through the passage of drugs into breast milk is determined by the following factors:

- The passage of the drug from the maternal blood into the milk
- The concentration of the drug in the milk
- The volume of milk sucked
- The pharmacokinetics of the drug in the infant, particularly its absorption and clearance
- The inherent toxicity of the drug

A list of such drugs can be found at the back of the BNF and should be consulted. The list includes common drugs such as the oral contraceptive, aspirin, atropine, ciprofloxin, penicillin and statins.

Self-assessment test

1 How does the normal ageing process affect renal function?
2 What are the three reasons for problems with medication in renal failure?
3 What two measurements are used to determine the degree of renal failure?

2 What are the four classifications of nephrotoxic drugs?

3 What is a therapeutic range?

4 What are phase I reactions?

5 What are phase II reactions?

6 What is enterohepatic circulation?

7 What three factors does hepatic clearance depend on?

8 If a drug is dependent on hepatic elimination, there are three factors to consider when prescribing for someone with liver disease. What are they?

9 List the factors that affect drug absorption in children.

10 When considering drug use in children, what age groupings should be used?

11 How can compliance be helped when considering prescribing for an elderly person?

12 Why is a lower starting dose sometimes used in the elderly?

13 Why is the elimination of drugs reduced in the elderly?

14 How does pregnancy alter distribution of drugs?

15 What is tetragenesis?

16 The passage of drugs into breast milk is determined by which five factors?

Reflective exercise

You have now read through and studied the contents of this chapter, and it is time for you to reflect on what you have learnt and consider how you are going to relate this to your prescribing practice. From what you have learnt, consider how this will influence what you prescribe. Will the information that you have learnt change any of the prescribing decisions that you thought you may have had previously, and if so, what, how and why?

References

British National Formulary (BNF). (2020). *BNF 79 (March)*. London: Pharmaceutical Press.

National Teratology Information Service (NTIS). Regional drug and therapeutic centre. Available at www.uktis.org.

NICE. (2008). *Early Identification and management of chronic kidney disease in adults in primary and secondary care.* London: NICE.

Reddy, B. (2006). Prescribing in older people. *Nurse Prescribing.* 4(9), 378–381.

The Kings Fund. (2013). *Polypharmacy and medicines optimization; making it safe and sound.* London: Kings Fund.

4 Clinical decision-making and assessment

Erica Smith and Natalie Ruscoe

Introduction

Clinical decision-making and effective history taking are imperative for safe prescribing. This chapter therefore covers the process and content of consultation with patients and some of the theoretical models of consultation which provide a framework for this. It discusses the process of history taking and the important aspect of clinical decision-making.

Learning objectives

By the end of this chapter, you will be able to

- Appreciate and understand the process and expected outcomes of consulting with a patient.
- Understand and consider how you will utilise some of the consultation and communication models into your own clinical area when undertaking a consultation.
- Consider the process of obtaining a history in a structure format and how this then informs your clinical decision-making for that patient.

Gathering information from a patient

In order to make sound clinical decisions, the practitioner must first gather as much information as possible from the patient in order to assist with the decision-making process. As experienced healthcare professionals, many non-medical prescribers have developed consultation and assessment skills prior to prescribing skills; however, these may need to be enhanced or refined as prescribing skills develop. Since 2006, qualified nurse independent and supplementary prescribers have been able to prescribe any medicine from the British National Formulary provided it is within their competence (Department of Health, 2006; Nursing and Midwifery Council, 2006). Nurses and other allied healthcare professionals may only prescribe however, once a full assessment has been undertaken, including a thorough history, such as medication and previous medical history (Health and Care Professions Council, 2019; Nursing and Midwifery Council, 2018).

Prescribing consultations have additional focus on achieving a diagnosis or differential diagnosis for which medications may be prescribed, with the diagnosis being in the history the majority of the time. In certain circumstances, it may be necessary to treat specific symptoms prior to a full diagnosis being reached, for example acute pain in patients who may not otherwise tolerate consultation and examination. Even in the most emergent of cases, there will need to be some element of consultation to determine the patients' complaint, previous medical history, any medications previously taken and allergies or contraindications to medications as a minimum.

Consultation with patients

Consultations will vary depending on the setting and circumstances within which they occur in. It may be the first time you meet a patient and they might need rapid treatment in an emergency department or you may know the patient well having reviewed them multiple times in clinic or general practice settings. These differences can alter the focus of the consultation (Figure 4.1).

Ideally a consultation will take place in a quiet, private space although in practice this may not always be possible with many hospital wards and departments only offering only curtains to protect patient's privacy. In circumstances where this becomes a barrier to gaining information, a more private location should be sought,

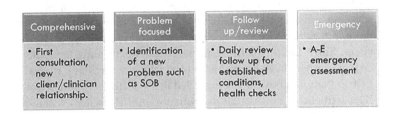

Figure 4.1 Focus of consultations.

and patients should be allowed to not answer questions if they feel uncomfortable about the possibility of being overheard (Douglas et al., 2009). In circumstances where a language barrier is present, attempts should be made to ensure this is overcome prior to the consultation commencing by offering appropriate translator or sign language interpreters as required.

First impressions are important and can have a significant influence on your subsequent relationship and the outcome of the encounter. Your demeanor, dress and attitude will influence your patient and how they take your advice, so ensure you introduce yourself and your role; ensure you check the patients' details, name, date of birth, and address. You should observe the patient's manner; do they appear distressed, observe for any non-verbal cues such as eye contact, changes in posture as they relax or become more closed.

A typical consultation involves gathering large amounts of information, inferring a diagnosis and formulating a management plan (Higgins, 2009). The importance of taking a comprehensive history cannot be overestimated; information should be gathered in a systematic, sensitive and professional manner (Crumbie, 2006). Practitioners with a deep and broad knowledge base are likely to pick up on more cues and question these during the deliberation phase of the decision-making process than novice practitioners. Despite technological advances in medicine, a thorough history and physical examination are still vital (Cotter, 2010). It is by the taking of a careful history that the good rapport essential for satisfactory management of any patient with any condition is achieved (Lee & Lin, 2008).

Consultation models

To assist with the development of consultation skills, there are numerous consultation models available. The best way to use consultation models is to read them all, see which you like and take the best out of each to develop your own model. Consultation models are not rules; they are learning aids to help you develop your own consultation skills. Having your own model ensures you have a system to rely on during the consultation process to achieve the best outcome for your patient. It also means you have a range of different techniques to use in difficult or differing consultations.

Pendelton, Schofield, Tate and Havelock (1984)

This patient-centred approach had two main characteristics. The first was to ensure effective communication between the doctor and the patient where they work together to define problems and decide on their management together. The second was a method of teaching in which the teacher and learner discover how to build on the learner's strengths to enhance his or her effectiveness (Pendelton et al., 2003). The revised 2003 model highlights six main points which they believe allow the achievement of understanding the illness from the patient perspective and shared information and decision-making. The key issues are to understand the problem and the patient; to share understanding, decisions and responsibility with the patient; to maintain the relationship and to do all of this within the allocated time (Pendelton et al., 2003). There is discussion about the potential tensions involved in patient-centred care. On the one hand, there is a moral imperative to provide information, empower patients and maximize patient choice as part of respecting patient autonomy. On the other hand, there is the medical imperative to improve health outcomes. The authors argue that fortuitously, the same consulting style maximizes both simultaneously (Pendelton et al., 2003).

Neighbour's model (1987)

The inner consultation model is one of the most well-recognised consultation models, which describes a five-stage model that should enable clinicians to consult more skilfully, more intuitively and more efficiently.

Neighbour proposed five checkpoints in the consultation:

1 ***Connecting***: Have we got rapport?
2 ***Summarising***: Could I demonstrate to the patient that I've sufficiently understood why he's come?

- The patient's reason for attending
- The patient's ideas and feelings, concerns and expectations are explored and I the patient has acknowledged adequately listening and eliciting of information from them
- The clinical process – assess, diagnose, explain, negotiate and agree

3 ***Handing over***: Has the patient accepted the management plan we have agreed?
4 ***Safety netting***: What if...? Clinical practice is the art of managing uncertainty:

- Predict what could happen if things go well
- Allow for an unexpected turn of events
- Plans and contingency plans

5 ***Housekeeping***: Am I in good condition for the next patient? (Neighbour, 1987).

Neighbour provides us with a model that is structured and easy to recall. Its five steps feel more achievable than Pendleton's seven steps. It is patient-centred but also attends to the doctor's feelings and tries to tackle the tricky areas that Byrne and Long identified as leading to dysfunctional consultations (Byrne & Long, 1976).

Byrne and Long (1976)

In 1976, Byrne and Long analysed more than 2,000 consultations and identified six logical phases to a consultation.

1 The doctor establishes a relationship with the patient.
2 The doctor attempts to discover or actually discovers the reasons for the patient's attendance.

3   The doctor conducts a verbal or physical examination or both.
4   The doctor and/or patient consider the condition.
5   The doctor and patient agree and detail further treatment or investigation if necessary.
6   The consultation is terminated (usually by the doctor).

Dysfunctional consultations usually fell down in phase 2 and/or 4.

Byrne and Long's study also analysed the range of verbal behaviours doctors used when talking to their patients. They described a spectrum ranging from a heavily doctor-dominated consultation, with any contribution from the patient as good as excluded, to a virtual monologue by the patient untrammelled by any input from the doctor. Between these extremes, they described a graduation of styles from closed information gathering to non-directive counselling, depending on whether the doctor was more interested in developing his or her own line of thought or the patient's (Byrne & Long, 1976).

Calgary-Cambridge communication skills framework

The Calgary-Cambridge guide to the medical interview (Silverman & Kurtz, 1996) was developed to describe effective physician–patient communication skills and to provide an evidence-based structure for their analysis and teaching. Whilst there are other tasks associated with the consultation, the guide is based on six communication skills tasks:

1   Initiating the consultation
2   Gathering information
3   Providing structure to the consultation
4   Building the relationship
5   Explanation and planning
6   Closing the consultation

While these tasks tend to be sequential, "building the relationship" and "providing structure" continue throughout the consultation. Within the six tasks, the guide itemises 77 separate communication skills. It has many similarities to Pendleton's earlier model. This is another five-stage model, which is very patient-centred. It incorporates the physical, psychological and social aspects of the consultation and is also very practical (Silverman et al., 2013).

The prescribing competency framework (RPS, 2016)

The Royal Pharmaceutical Society provides a framework for all prescribers in collaboration with all prescribing professions across the UK and sets out the competencies expected of all prescribers to support safe prescribing (Royal Pharmaceutical Society, 2016). In this they describe the competencies required as part of the consultation process which highlights six key roles of the consultation:

1 Assess the patient.
2 Consider the options.
3 Reach a shared decision.
4 Prescribe.
5 Provide information.
6 Monitor and review.

Although multiple consultation models are available, whichever is used it is vital to remember that good clinician–patient communication is vital and especially important when new medications are prescribed, since patients frequently misunderstand information or have difficulty reading medication labels (Davis et al., 2006). The ability of clinicians to communicate effectively about medication is vital as patients' beliefs about medication and their understanding of their diagnosis which may influence their adherence to treatment. (This framework is also covered in full in Chapter 1.)

History taking

Irrespective of which consultation method is used, there are common key information requirements.

Patient complaint or presenting complaint/ condition – The reason the patient has requested consultation best described in one sentence and as the patient says it.

History of patient complaint – This gives the opportunity to explore the patients' perspective of the problem you should avoid leading questions and allow the patient to give as much information as possible. Once a patient has been interrupted, they rarely introduce new issues (Gask & Usherwood, 2002). All symptoms disclosed should be questioned fully in turn in order to get full details of the symptom, before moving on to the next. In order to gain a better understanding of symptoms, there is a range of mnemonics that can be used. For example, SOCRATES is an extremely useful tool for enquiring about pain and widely cited in medical literature (Colledge et al., 2010; Douglas et al., 2009; Wyatt & Graham, 2012).

S – Site

O – Onset

C – Character

R – Radiation

A – Associated symptoms

T – Time intensity relationship (does it come and go or is it constant)

E – Exacerbating and relieving factors

S – Severity

Similarly other mnemonics can be used or modified to gain further information about a number of symptoms. Once a symptom has been explored using questions to clarify information or gain further information, the cardinal-associated symptoms which relate to the system being discussed should be explored; for example, patients who attend complaining of shortness of breath should always be specifically asked about cough, sputum, haemoptysis, wheeze, chest pain, oedema, paroxysmal dyspnoea and orthopnoea.

It is also useful to try and determine a baseline in terms of function and ability: when was the patient last well? Or how much can the patient normally do for themselves, and how far can they normally walk without chest pain or shortness of breath? In some instances, it is important to try and determine what has happened since the initial presenting complaint; for example, a patient who presents with a three-month history of shortness of breath is likely to have had some treatment or investigations already, and therefore, their management will be considerably different from the patient who started feeling short of breath on the day or day before they attend. It is important to try and determine what a patient means by a phrase or word as this is not always necessarily the same as your understanding of the same phrase; this is particularly important with terms such as dizzy; for example, do they mean dizzy or presyncope.Sick is also sometimes used to describe vomiting, but they just mean generally unwell andlethargic.

It can also be useful to ask questions during the history of patient complaint which are covered in other areas of the history, for example asking about smoking in patients with ischaemic heart disease or asking about anticoagulation in patients presenting with head injuries.

On occasions, it may be necessary to gain this information partly or wholly from others: a patient with advanced dementia may be unable to explain why he or she is now presenting, and similarly a patient who has had a loss of consciousness or seizure may be able to provide part of the history but have no recollection of other events. In such circumstances, bystander history can be vital in trying to determine what has actually happened and can have a significant impact on the diagnosis and management for that patient.

Past medical history (PMH): PMH may be relevant to the presenting complaint and ask about previous illnesses, operations and injuries, and when these were. These can be verified by medical notes, electronic history systems and patients' relatives. Current pregnancy, planning for a pregnancy and breastfeeding will also need to be explored in women of childbearing age as certain drugs may need to be avoided.

Drug history: Ask about prescribed drugs and any other medications. Include over-the-counter remedies and alternative medicine treatments, particularly herbal or homeopathic remedies, laxatives, analgesics and vitamins or mineral supplements. If possible, ask to see the medication and/or a recent prescription list. Note the name of each drug, the dose, dosage regime and the duration of treatment, along with any significant side effects. Check for any change in dose, new medications or recently discontinued medications.

Ask patients to describe how and when they take their medications and give them the opportunity to admit they do not take all their medicines as prescribed as this is common in practice (Elwyn et al., 2003; Latter, 2010); sometimes, this can be evident when medications they have with them have been dispensed months or even years ago, or if they are not collecting repeat prescriptions. Concordance can be assessed with the following questions: Are any medications causing side effects? Changed doses or stopped due to effects? Do you stop taking when feeling better? Or do you stop taking when feeling worse?

Allergies and reactions: Ask if your patient has ever had an allergic reaction to medications. Clarify exactly what patients mean by an allergy. Enquire specifically before prescribing an antibiotic, especially penicillin. Ask about other allergies such as foodstuffs, animal hair, pollen or metals.

Family history: Use open questions such as "are there any illnesses that run in your family?" The presenting complaint may direct you to a specific line of enquiry. A patient presenting with ischaemic heart disease, for example, should be asked directly about any family history of ischaemic heart disease; where appropriate, ask about any young sudden deaths in the family. Document illness in first-degree relative, that is parents, siblings, and children, where these relatives are deceased try and determine a cause of death for them.

Social history: The social history helps you to understand the context of the patient's life and possible relevant factors. Ask about occupation, diet, exercise, travel, smoking, alcohol and recreational drug use, along with home circumstances and sexual health.

Systems review: A systems review that occurs at the end of a history can uncover symptoms that may have been forgotten. Ask "is there anything else you would like to tell me about?" It can be done in a head-to-toe fashion in order to ensure no symptoms are missed.

Data gained during the consultation can and should be verified; physical examination and investigations together with blister packs of medication, repeat prescription, community pharmacist documentation, general practitioner (GP) or other medical records can all add to the information gained.

When you have all the information required, share your thoughts and conclusions with the patient in language which is clear and concise and that they are able to understand. Ensure that the patient has understood the information but also that he or she agrees with any planned treatment as there is no point prescribing a medication which will not be taken. Ensure they understand any safety netting you have discussed and that the course of illness may change and that they should seek further review if this happens. Always offer an opportunity for the patient to ask questions and clarify anything that they have not understood. If they ask questions you are unable to answer, ensure that you are honest with them and explain that you will need to seek information from colleagues or other source and get back to them with this information.

Clinical decision-making theories

Once the information has been gathered, then clinicians must make a decision on a management plan for their patient; this may include the need to prescribe or not to prescribe medication. There are a number of decision-making theories which describe how these decisions can be arrived at. The most commonly used is the hypothetical-deductive reasoning model where clinicians build up a hypothesis of possible diagnosis and use cues to confirm or reduce the likelihood of such hypothesis being correct (Elstein & Schwarz, 2002). Other clinical decision-making methods include pattern recognition where decisions are based on the fact that these symptoms and presentations have been seen previously by the clinician and treated successfully in a certain way; therefore, treatment is based on the previous experience (Evans, 2005). Similarly intuition has been described as a clinical decision-making theory often described as a "gut feeling" and based on experience and thought to be a subconscious process of decision-making (Buckingham & Adams, 2000). In reality, clinicians are likely to use a combination of decision-making practices in order to process information and decide on management plans for patients.

Conclusion

Prescribing decisions are a complex task and can only be made once a thorough history has been taken. Picking up on and responding to patients' cues is an important part of taking a history; it is important not to miss these cues which can be verbal or non-verbal in nature and may include changes in posture, eye contact and tone of voice (Gask & Usherwood, 2002). Good clinical knowledge and experience are necessary in order to recognise and investigate all the cues, which can then form the basis of sound clinical decisions. Once these decisions are made, good communication skills are required to share information, which is likely to lead to better and more appropriate use of medication (Heath, 2003; Hobden, 2006; Segal, 2007). The consultation should be used to enhance the relationship with patients increasing their trust in you and giving them the information required to promote their own health, even when this means that the consultation has not led to a prescription of medication sharing advice, including the advice that antibiotics are not required for viral illnesses is equally important as writing a prescription when one is indicated.

Self-assessment test

1   Name two consultation models and consider how you would implement these in your own clinical practice.
2   What are the six communication skills in the Calgary-Cambridge model?
3   What are the eight stages of history taking?

Reflective exercise

You have now read through and studied the contents of this chapter, and it is time for you to reflect on what you have learnt and consider how you are going to relate this to your prescribing practice. From what you have learnt, consider how this will influence what you prescribe. Will the information that you have learnt change any of the prescribing decisions that you thought you may have had previously, and if so, what, how and why?

References

Buckingham, C., & Adams, A. (2000). Classifying clinical decision making: interpreting nursing intuition, heuristics and medical diagnosis. *Journal of Advanced Nursing.* 32(4), 990–999.

Byrne, P., & Long, B. (1976). *Doctors talking to patients.* London: HMSO.

Colledge, N., Walker, B., & Ralston, S. (2010). *Davidson's principles & practice of medicine* (21st ed.). Edinburgh: Churchill Livingstone Elsevier.

Cotter, L. (2010). History and examination of the cardiovascular system. *Medicine.* 38(7), 344–347.

Crumbie, A. (2006). Taking a history. In: M. Walsh, ed. *Nurse practitioners: clinical skills and professional issues.* Edinburgh: Butterworth Heinmann, pp. 14–27.

Davis, T.C., Wolf, M., Bass, P., Thompson, J.A., Tilson, H.H., Neuberger, M., & Parker, R. (2006). Literacy and misunderstanding prescriptin drug labels. *Annals of Internal Medicine.* 145(12), 887–894.

Department of Health. (2006). *Improving patients' access to medicine: A guide to implementing nurse and pharmacist independent prescribing within the NHS in England.* London: Department of Health.

Douglas, G., Nicol, F., & Robertson, C. (2009). *Macleod's clinical examination* (12th ed.). Edinburgh: Churchill Livingstone Elsevier.

Elstein, A., & Schwarz, A. (2002). Clinical problem solving and diagnositic decision making: selective review of the cognitive literature. *British Medical Journal.* 324(7339), 729–732.

Elwyn, G., Edwards, A., & Britten, N. (2003). "Doing prescribing": how doctors can be more effective. *British Medical Journal.* 327, 864–867.

Evans, C. (2005). Clinical decision making theories: patient assessment in A&E. *Emergency Nurse.* 13(5), 16–19.

Gask, L., & Usherwood, T. (2002). ABC of psychological medicine: the consultation. *BMJ.* 324(7353), 1567–1569.

Health and Care Professions Council. (2019). *Standards for prescribing* [Online]. Available at https://www.hcpc-uk.org/standards/standards-relevant-to-education-and-training/standards-for-prescribing/. Accessed 7 May 2020.

Higgins, R. (2009). Abdominal assessment and diagnosis of appendicitis. *Emergency Nurse.* 16(9), 22–24.

Kemp, R., Hayward, P., Applewhaite, G., Everitt, B., & David, A. (1997). Compliance therapy in psychotic patients: randomised controlled trial. *British Medical Journal.* 312, 345–349.

Latter, S. (2010). Promoting concordance in prescribing interactions. In: M. Courtney & M. Griffiths, eds. *Independent and supplementary prescribing. An essential guide.* Cambridge: Cambridge University Press, pp. 107–119.

Latter, S., Maben, J., Myall, M., & Young, A. (2007). Perecptions and practice of concordance in nurses' prescribing consultations: findings from a national questionnaire survey and case studies of practice in England. *International Journal of Nursing Studies.* 44, 9–18.

Lawson, M.T. (2002). Nurse practitioner and physician communication styles. *Applied Nursing Research.* 15(2), 60–66.

Lee, Y.Y., & Lin, J.L. (2008). Linking patients' trust in physicians to health outcomes. *British Journal of Hospital Medicine.* 69(1), 42–46.

Neighbour, R. (1987). *The inner consultation.* Oxford: Radcliffe Medical Press.

Nursing and Midwifery Council. (2006). *Standards for proficiency for nurse and midwife prescribers.* London: Nursing and Midwifery Council.

Nursing and Midwifery Council. (2018). *Realising professionalism: standards for education and training part 3: Standards for prescribing programmes* [Online]. Available at https://www.nmc.org.uk/globalassets/sitedocuments/education-standards/programme-standards-prescribing.pdf. Accessed 7 May 2020.

Pendelton, D., Schofield, T., Tate, P., & Havelock, P. (2003). *The new consultation: developing doctor-patient communication.* New York: Oxford University Press.

Royal Pharmaceutical Society. (2016). *Prescribing framework a competency framework for all Prescribers* [Online]. Available at https://www.rpharms.com/Portals/0/RPS%20document%20library/Open%20access/Professional%20standards/Prescribing%20competency%20framework/prescribing-competency-framework.pdf?ver=2019-02-13-163215-030. Accessed 3 May 2020.

Silverman, J., & Kurtz, S. (1996). The Calgary-Cambridge referenced observation guides: an aid to defining the curriculum and organizing the teaching in communication training programmes. *Medical education.* 30(2), 83–89.

Silverman, J., Kurtz, S., & Draper, J. (2013). *Skills for communicating with patients* (3rd ed.). New York: CRC Press.

Wyatt, J., & Graham, C. (2012). *Oxford handbook of emergency medicine* (4th ed.). Oxford: Oxford University Press.

5 Legal, professional, policy and ethical aspects of prescribing

Natalie Ruscoe and Erica Smith

Introduction

Legal, ethical and professional issues are integral principles of all healthcare professionals' roles, and awareness and understanding of these are essential. This chapter explores these principles we not only know and understand them but can also apply them to our practice.

Learning outcomes

At the end of this chapter, you will be able to

1   Understand the professional aspects of prescribing.
2   Understand the legal aspects of prescribing.
3   Understand the ethical aspects of prescribing.

Professional aspects of non-medical prescribing

Accountability and who we are accountable to are common terms associated with being a healthcare professional. Accountability relates to being responsible for one's actions (or omissions), and by being held to account, we may be required to explain or justify those actions to others. As nurses and allied health professionals, due to our professional roles and responsibilities, we are accountable to many: we are accountable to our patients, the public, our employers and ultimately our professional regulators (see Figure 5.1). With a strong link to our legal and ethical responsibilities, professional issues are often not seen in isolation.

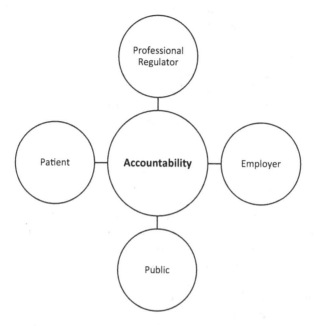

Figure 5.1 Accountability responsibilities.

Professional regulator: As healthcare professionals, we are regulated by our professional body, the Nursing and Midwifery Council (NMC) for nurses and allied health professionals and the Health and Care Professions Council (HCPC). Both regulatory bodies provide a code of professional conduct, advising practitioners of their professional requirements and standards for performance (HCPC, 2016; NMC, 2018a), and as such this offers a certain level of assurance to the public, a level of quality that they can expect from a registered practitioner providing treatment or care. It is the role of the regulators to hold those on their register to account for any actions or omissions that fall below these standards, thus protecting the public. Whilst this may sound punitive in nature, accountability is not just about blame but indeed should be used to evidence safe and effective practice.

As a non-medical prescriber, it is important that we consider our accountability and how this role may impact it. Both regulators (HCPC, 2016; NMC, 2018a) advise practitioners of their responsibilities such as working within their limits of competence and scope and practice, working to the best available evidence base, record keeping and managing/identifying risk. Prescribing, whether independently or supplementary, increases our scope of practice and as such our levels of responsibility, and with this responsibility comes accountability. Through standards of education and practice set by both regulatory bodies (HCPC, 2019; NMC, 2018b), only practitioners who have successfully completed the required educational training will have the additional prescribing annotation added to their professional register. With competency being determined through the Royal Pharmaceutical Society (2016) competency framework; this level of competency must be maintained throughout the practitioner's prescribing practice and is a benchmark for our practice – a standard for our accountability to be measured against.

Employer: Most healthcare practitioners will be employed within a healthcare organisation, although it is acknowledged that some will be self-employed. For those employed, they are also held to account via their contract of employment. An employment contract is considered to be binding in law and as such has obligations for both parties. Through vicarious liability, our employers ultimately will be liable for any mistakes or errors that we make, provided these occurred whilst acting in the course of your employment. For non-medical prescribers, this would include prescribing when part of your job description and role.

While employers have a duty of care to their employees, importantly employees also have a duty to their employers. These duties include taking reasonable care whilst undertaking business on behalf of your employer, but also it includes a duty to obey reasonable instructions from your employer (Dimond, 2011). It is this through employer policies and procedures where employees could be held accountable. A breach in adhering to policies and procedures could lead to disciplinary action, and should a patient come to harm, other proceedings such as civil or criminal prosecutions alongside these could also be initiated. Therefore, as a non-medical prescriber, it is important that procedures and guidelines are followed, in line with best practice and any such deviation can be clearly justified.

Public: Through the laws of our society, non-medical prescribers can also be held to account. Whilst the vast majority of healthcare professionals seek to live both their personal and professional lives in a law-abiding way, any such deviation from this, for example where a healthcare professional knowingly causes harm, would result in criminal proceedings like any other citizen. It would most likely also lead to fitness to practice investigations and sanctions with their regulatory body. As a healthcare professional and non-medical prescriber, whilst abiding by the laws set down in society, we must also work within the legislation that exists in terms of the prescription, supply and administration of medicines as well as other health and social care legislation. While poor standards of practice or clinical negligence claims in relation to healthcare professionals are typically dealt with through the professional regulators and the civil courts, in the most severe of cases of clinical negligence, usually where the negligence has resulted in the death of a patient, criminal prosecutions may also be considered.

Patient: Patients trust healthcare professionals to care for them and treat them, to relieve symptoms, to improve quality of life and, where possible, to cure them of their illnesses or injuries. As a non-medical prescriber, the ability to complete an episode of care from assessment, examination to treatment can be extremely satisfying and also provides huge benefits to patient care. During care or treatment, patients may access many healthcare professionals, and each has a duty of care to that patient, being accountable for that care or treatment provided. If a patient perceives that their treatment falls below an acceptable level, for any reason, they can hold that practitioner to account. In relation to prescribing, their concerns may include issues such as diagnosis or misdiagnosis of a condition and its subsequent treatment, errors or omissions, poor communication around treatment options, monitoring or adverse reactions. Patients can raise a concern or make a complaint through your employer and can also refer their concerns about you to your professional regulator, both of whom are obligated to review and investigate the concerns raised. Patients can also hold you to account through the civil courts if clinical negligence is alleged.

Legal aspects of non-medical prescribing

The legal aspects of non-medical prescribing can be considered in terms of the laws that govern prescribing and medicines, and the civil and criminal systems that protect the public.

Legislation: Non-medical prescribing is regulated by the law, and who can prescribe and what can be prescribed is enshrined within these acts of parliament and laws. The main legislations related to medicines and prescribing are the Medicines Act 1968, Human Medicines Regulations 2012, Misuse of Drugs Act 1971 and Misuse of Drugs Regulations 2001.

The Medicinal Products (Prescription by Nurses etc) Act 1992 was the first legislative change made to existing legislation within the Medicines Act 1968 to give non-medical practitioners specific rights to prescribe. The Medicines Act 1968 and the Human Medicines Regulations 2012 and its amendments consolidate much of the law concerning medicinal products and prescribing. Between these and the Misuse of Drugs Act 1971, the legislation on the supply, storage and administration of medicines, with the latter also focusing more on controlled drugs, captures the main legal principles. As prescription-only medicines (POMs) were only initially legally prescribed by a doctor, dentist or veterinarian, amendments have continued to be made to the legislation to allow non-medical prescribers to be able to legally prescribe. The term "appropriate practitioner" is often used within the legislation to describe healthcare professionals who are legally trained to prescribe medicines. Prescribing amongst non-medical professionals continues to expand, with advanced paramedics being the latest to be granted prescribing rights in 2018 (College of Paramedics, 2018). A current list of non-medical prescribers who are legally able to prescribe can be seen in Table 5.1.

The Medicines Act 1968 classifies medicinal products into categories: general sales list (GSL), pharmacy (P) and prescription-only medicines (POM) with the legislation discussed above also stipulating the legal requirements in terms of writing prescriptions,

Table 5.1 Current non-medical prescribers

Independent prescribing	Supplementary prescribing
Nurses and midwives	Nurses and midwives
Pharmacists	Pharmacists
Chiropodists/podiatrists	Chiropodists/podiatrists
Paramedics	Paramedics
Physiotherapists	Physiotherapists
Therapeutic radiographers	Therapeutic radiographers
	Dieticians
	Diagnostic radiographers

providing guidance on the manufacturing, licencing and supply of medications. Non-medical prescribers need to be aware of their legal obligations when prescribing medications and completing a prescription to ensure compliance, as breaches of these laws could lead the prescriber being held accountable. The legal requirements in relation to prescription writing include the following:

- Legible writing
- Being indelible
- Signing and dating the prescription
- The patient's name and address
- The address of the prescriber (practice area)
- An indication of the type of prescriber
- The age and date of birth should also be stated preferably in all patients but is a legal requirement in those under 12 years old (NICE, 2020a)

The prescribing of controlled drugs (Schedules 2 and 3) has additional prescribing writing requirements to the above list:

- The total quantity to be supplied must be documented in words and figures
- The type of medicines/preparation (e.g. tablet, liquid)
- Strength of drug and dose to be administered (NICE, 2020b)

By law, if the legal requirements are not met within a prescription chart, it cannot be dispensed. More specifically to controlled drugs, the Misuse of Drugs Act 1971 lists and classifies controlled drugs and has powers within the Act, which means possession and supply without a prescription is a criminal offence. The Misuse of Drugs Regulations 2001 permits the supply, prescription and administration of these medicines, dividing the controlled drugs into five schedules (see Table 5.2), with each having its own requirements in relation to supply, possession, prescribing and record keeping. Therefore, as a prescriber, it is important to know what requirements are required for any controlled drugs prescribed.

Within non-medical prescribing, there are some disparities between healthcare professionals prescribing rights including

Table 5.2 Drugs schedules, Misuse of Drugs Regulations 2001

Schedule 1	*Home Office authority required*
Schedule 2	Includes diamorphine, morphine, pethidine, glutethimide, amphetamine
	Subject to full-controlled drug regulations including additional prescription requirements
Schedule 3	Barbiturates, buprenorphine, diethylpropion, midazolam, temazepam, tramadol
	Similar to Schedule 2 with some exceptions (e.g. Temazepam is not subject to additional prescription requirements; tramadol and midazolam are exempt from safe custody requirements, but invoices need to be kept for a minimum of two years)
	Note: Gabapentin and pregabalin became a Schedule 3 controlled drug in April 2019. These are now subject to additional prescription requirements but are exempt from safe custody requirements
Schedule 4	Part 1 – Benzodiazepines: diazepam, lorazepam (except temazepam and midazolam) and zopiclone
	Part 2 – Androgenic and anabolic steroids
	Additional prescription requirements do not apply, and Schedule 4 drugs are not subject to safe custody requirements.
Schedule 5	Includes preparations of certain controlled drugs which due to their strength are exempt from nearly all controlled drug requirements other than retention of invoices for two years

Source: NICE. (2020b); Dimond. (2011)

controlled drugs. Whilst in England, nurses and pharmacists are permitted to prescribe schedules 2, 3, 4 and 5 controlled drugs with a few exceptions and can independently prescribe any drug for any condition (licenced or unlicensed) if competent to do so, physiotherapists and paramedics can only prescribe unlicensed medications via supplementary prescribing and an agreed clinical management plan (Chartered Society of Physiotherapists, 2018; College of Paramedics, 2018). Controlled drugs for independent prescribing physiotherapists are limited to morphine (oral or injectable), fentanyl (transdermal), diazepam, dihydrocodeine, lorazepam, oxycodone hydrochloride and temazepam (oral). Podiatrists have a further limited number of controlled drugs, such as diazepam, dihydrocodeine, lorazepam and temazepam (oral), and to date, paramedics are not able to prescribe controlled drugs as an amendment is required to the Misuse of Drugs Regulations. It is therefore essential that each non-medical prescriber fully understands their legal standing in relation to their profession.

Civil law: As healthcare professionals and prescribers, we owe a duty of care to our patients and clients that we treat and care for. When care falls below an acceptable standard, and harm occurs due to negligence, patients can hold the practitioner delivering that care to account. Civil law and negligence are covered by the law of tort, and unlike the high burden of proof required within criminal cases (beyond reasonable doubt), civil law rests on the balance of probability (Avery, 2013) and often seeks to compensate the victim via financial redress. While many cases of clinical negligence will be covered via vicarious liability for those employed and acting within their agreed job roles and boundaries, it is essential that professional indemnity insurance is also held (Brack, 2014; NMC, 2018a).

Clinical negligence can be caused by errors in practice, actions or omissions; such as things that you did or did not do. These errors, while often unintentional, may have resulted in a delayed diagnosis or misdiagnosis, or a failure to perform a procedure correctly, or a failure to sufficiently warn a patient about risks, affecting the choice made by patients or by providing incorrect information (Davey et al., 2017). Healthcare professionals and prescribers are required to meet a minimum standard of care, and falling below this standard could lead to negligent practice. If this negligence in practice causes harm, then a patient could accuse you of clinical negligence and claim compensation.

For clinical negligence claims to be successful, claimants need to prove that

- A duty of care was owed to them by the defendant (the healthcare professional).
- The duty of care was breached by negligence/care below the minimum standard.
- The breach was caused by the defendant and resulted in harm to the claimant (usually the patient).

While the landmark "snail in the ale" case *Donoghue v Stevenson* [1932] established and defined duty of care, within health where practitioners are caring for and treating patients, it is easy for patients to demonstrate that a duty of care exists. However, demonstrating that there was a breach in this duty requires causation. Causation, also known as the "but for" test, means that but for the actions/omissions of the defendant, the claimant would not have been harmed. Not all breaches in care cause harm, and without this, a practitioner is not held liable for negligence (Davey et al., 2017). Therefore, the claimant must prove both that their actions/omissions were negligent and caused harm as a result. Breaches in duty of care caused by negligence can be complicated cases, but key landmark cases have been applied over the years to determine if negligence has occurred.

Bolam v Friern Hospital Management Committee [1957], often referred to as the "Bolam test", found that a healthcare professional cannot be found negligent if they act in accordance with an accepted body of practice that is supported by medical opinion. In this case, the claimant, Mr Bolam, was being treated for depression with electroconvulsive therapy. During treatment, no muscle relaxants or manual restraints were used, and as a result of treatment, Mr Bolam sustained a fracture to his pelvis. The claimant alleged that this fracture was a result of negligence, but the hospital treating argued that their practice was in line with what other professionals also did and subsequently were found not to be negligent. Key findings from the case recognised that negligence occurs when standards fall below those that are reasonable what a "reasonably competent" person would do. It also recognised that more than one method of practice may be acceptable but should be in accordance with what the judge deciding over the case called "a responsible body of medical men skilled in that particular art" – Judge McNair.

Importantly, within clinical negligence, inexperience does not count as a defence or an excuse. Within prescribing, by successfully completing the educational programme, you will have proved yourself as competent and should therefore work above the minimum acceptable standard of practice expected of any prescriber with Griffith and Dowey (2019, p. 65) stating that a "patient is entitled to receive the accepted standard of care whoever provides it". Equally, they would also argue that obeying orders is unlikely to be a successful defence as all healthcare professionals have individual accountability for their actions.

In recent years, there has been some criticism of the Bolam test, with some believing that the courts should take a more active role in scrutinising the standards of care being provided, rather than relying on healthcare professionals (Bartlett & Eaton, 2019). The case of *Bolitho v City and Hackney Health Authority* [1998] highlighted this. Whilst the case was found in favour of the defendant (that negligence had not occurred), during the House of Lords review of the case, the Bolam test was discussed and they added that the courts need to be satisfied that an accepted body of practice can withstand objective scrutiny and can demonstrate a "logical basis". This key point being made clear to healthcare professions within this judgement is that if the accepted body of practice could not withstand logical assessment, then a judge is entitled to decide otherwise.

With clinical guidelines and national standards/polices from institutions such as National Institute for Health and Care Excellence (NICE) increasingly being used to set benchmarks for reasonable standards of care, non-medical prescribers need to ensure that they work within their scope of practice and, importantly, within the guidelines that demonstrate this acceptable body of practice that would be able to withstand scrutiny from the courts.

Criminal law: The death of a patient through gross negligence may be the point where the civil law of negligence crosses over into the criminal law systems. Griffith and Dowie (2019) report that in the post Mid Staffordshire NHS Foundation Trust and the Winterbourne View Hospital inquiries, more emphasis has been placed on holding individuals and organisations to account, to restore public confidence, and cases that may have previously have been dealt with purely by regulators, employers and civil courts may also now be coming before the criminal courts, under the charge of manslaughter by gross negligence.

Criminal conviction needs to be proven beyond reasonable doubt (Avery, 2013). As the purpose of the criminal justice system is punitive, a higher burden of proof is required. According to the Crown Prosecution Service (2019), the offence of gross negligence manslaughter is committed where the death (of a patient) is a result of a grossly negligent act or omission on the part of the defendant (the practitioner). The case of *R v Adomako* [1994] was a significant case in relation to this issue and involved an anaesthetist who during an eye operation failed to recognise in a timely manner that the ventilatory tubing had become disconnected from the patient. This subsequently led to the cardiac arrest and death of the patient. The case found that the defendant had fallen far below the required standard and as such was negligent in their practice. Moreover, it was also argued that any reasonable doctor should have recognised this issue quickly, and, in this case, the defendant's conduct was deemed so bad that it amounted to a criminal act. Therefore, criminal prosecution could be considered for manslaughter by gross negligence if the care or treatment that is delivered to a patient is so poor or inadequate, so "truly exceptionally bad" that it results in their death (Williams, 2018).

While the criminal prosecution of healthcare professionals for manslaughter by gross negligence is very rare, in recent years, high-profile cases such as the Dr Bawa-Garba case (*R v Bawa-Garba* [2015]; *Bawa-Garba v GMC* [2018]), which resulted in the death of a six-year-old boy, have led to some concern within the healthcare professions and have brought negligence by gross negligence and professional regulation to the forefront of our minds.

Ethical aspects of non-medical prescribing

Ethics can be described as a system of principles, often linked to rights, wrongs and morals and can be depicted by a series of theories such as consequentialism, deontology and biomedical ethics. Within this section, biomedical ethics and the four ethical principles based on the work of Beauchamp and Childress (2013) will be explored: beneficence, non-maleficence, autonomy and justice. These four principles intertwined with our professional and legal obligations form a basis in which we practice as healthcare professionals and non-medical prescribers.

Beneficence: Beneficence can be described as the act of doing good for our patients. As healthcare professionals, we have an obligation to do good, putting the welfare of patients at the centre of the decisions we make (Davey et al., 2017), and this is linked closely to our professional obligations and codes of practice (HCPC, 2016; NMC, 2018a). However, Beauchamp and Childress (2013) point out that to do good takes active steps, not merely refraining from causing harm. Therefore, with non-medical prescribing, we must use our skills and knowledge to improve patient care and alleviate symptoms, improving quality of life where possible.

Non-maleficence: The principle of non-maleficence means we should not cause harm to others. Whilst linked to the principle of beneficence, non-maleficence is often a principle that clearly resonates to healthcare professionals, with our intention to do good rather than harm. Non-maleficence also links to negligence and standards of care (Beauchamp & Childress, 2013). If we do harm, even unintentionally, this could be due to a negligent act, or when care or treatment has fallen below the standards expected. An example of this may be where harm is caused by prescribing a medication where there is known interaction or contraindication which results in complications for the patient. However, the principle of non-maleficence whilst aiming to do no harm is also linked to minimising harm because when prescribing medications, we often aim to alleviate symptoms and treat disease, but these medications themselves do not come without some risk. Some medications may come with quite significant side effects, so when considering their use, the benefits (of doing good) need to outweigh that risk of harm.

***Autonomy*:** Autonomy relates to respect for individuals and their right to choose, their right to self-determination and self-rule. As healthcare professionals, we have a responsibility to provide patients with the necessary information and to support them to make their own informed decisions. It is not the responsibility of healthcare professional to make decision for those capable of making their own choices. Patients with capacity have the right to make their own choices, regardless of whether we agree with them or not. Patients have the right to refuse treatments and should be supported to make choices on treatment options where more than one exists based on the evidence available. As healthcare professionals, we need to respect the autonomous choices made by patients, because to be truly autonomous means you have chosen your own path, free from controlling interference (Beauchamp & Childress, 2013).

Autonomy, however, can be a complex concept and is linked to informed consent and mental capacity. The Department of Health (2009, p. 9) states that for consent to be valid, it must "…be given voluntarily by an appropriately informed person, who has the capacity to consent to the intervention in question…" The Mental Capacity Act 2005 defines that a person lacks capacity if they are "…unable to make a decision for themselves because of an impairment or disturbance in the functioning of their mind or brain…" which can be temporary or permanent. The Mental Capacity Act 2005 therefore determines how healthcare professionals should act when treating patients. If patients are deemed to have capacity, they must be able to understand the information given to them, retain that information for a long enough period of time to weight it up as part of making the decision, and communicate their wishes in some form or another (Department of Health, 2009; Mental Capacity Act, 2005). If a patient is able to do this, they have the necessary capacity to make that decision. This may relate to refusing treatments (e.g. anticoagulation for atrial fibrillation despite the risk of stroke), life-sustaining treatments such as chemotherapy or blood products based on religious beliefs. Therefore, with the presumption that patients have the capacity to make their own decisions, consent for treatment is required and patients need to be supported to make an informed choice, with their choices being respected to promote the principle of autonomy.

Where patients lack the capacity to make their own decisions, treatment decisions can be made by healthcare professionals in line with the patient's best interests, by someone with parental responsibility, by someone authorised to do so under a Lasting Power of Attorney (LPA) or occasionally through the courts. With children, the core principle of the Children Act 1989 is the child's welfare and their protection. To provide consent for a child, parental responsibility is required. An adult is defined in the Children Act 1989 as a person above 18 years of age. Although children aged 16–17 years are presumed to be competent to give consent, children less than 16 years of age can be considered slightly more complex. In children less than 16 years of age, if a child shows sufficient understanding and maturity with regard to their treatment, they can consent for themselves; this is termed "Gillick competence" and was the guidance provided following the legal challenge found in *Gillick v West Norfolk* and *Wisbech Area Health Authority* [1985]. The "Gillick competence" in essence advocates autonomy for children, but importantly children under 16 years cannot simply refuse treatment and parental consent can be used for children who are incapable of consent or are refusing treatment that is in their best interests.

All healthcare professionals and non-medical prescribers who will be treating adults or children need to ensure they have a clear understanding of this relevant legislation and guidance, to promote autonomy and also to know when intervention on a patient's best interest is required.

Justice: Justice within biomedical ethics relates to what is fair and reasonable. It relates to treating patients in a fair and equitable manner. As the national health service (NHS) faces unprecedented demands, justice and the fair allocation of resources is often considered a true ethical dilemma. With suggestions of rationing and postcode lotteries, some would argue that justice can sometimes be the less dominating of the principles (Johnston & Bradbury, 2016) and resources that are finite related to funding and medicines can cause significant conflict. As non-medical prescribers, using guidance from national institutions such as NICE and local prescribing formularies will hopefully help to promote the fair allocation of resources amongst patients.

Consent

Any adult has the right in law to be consented about any treatment that they are to receive or undergo. They should not be touched without consent, and if they are without consent or other lawful justification, then the person has the right of action in the civil courts of suing for trespass to the person.

The fact that consent has been given will normally prevent a successful action for trespass. However, it may not prevent an action of negligence arising on the grounds that a breach of duty of care has occurred following the consent from the person being given.

To be valid, consent must be given voluntarily by a mentally competent person without any duress or fraud. There are different forms of consent and these are express, which can be either written or verbal, and implied. As far as the law is concerned, there is no specific requirement that consent for treatment should be given in any particular way. They are all equally valid. However, they vary considerably in their value as evidence in providing that consent was given. Consent in writing is far the best form of evidence and is therefore the preferred method of obtaining the consent of the patient when any procedure where some risk is contemplated.

The Department of Health updated its guidance on consent to examination and treatment in 2001 and produced two publications: a reference guide to the principles on consent to examination and treatment and a good practice in consent implementation guide. The guidance has also been amended in line with the Mental Capacity Act.

Consent, it should be noted, is not a defence to an offence of causing actual bodily harm under the Offences Against the Person Act 1861.

The forms of consent to examination and treatment that are contained in the Department of Health implementation guidance (DH, 2001) require the health professional providing the treatment to discuss with the patient the benefits of the treatment and also any serious or frequently occurring risks associated with it and also identify any additional procedures which may be necessary, including the possibility of a blood transfusion or other specific procedures.

Consent is not simply a signature on a form; it is the result of a process of communication between patient and professional that may result in the patient signing a form, which is evidence that the patient agree to the proposed treatment.

As with other forms of treatment, patient consent is required for the administration of medication. For that consent to be valid, patients must be provided with significant information about the products prescribed, including information about known side effects, to allow them to make informed decisions. They should be made aware of the risks of the medication prescribed and any alternatives available. The amount of information patients need depends upon a range of factors including the diagnosis, the prognosis, the type of medication proposed, the level of risk associated with it and the amount of information the patient is willing or able to accept.

Nurse and allied health professional prescribers need to have up-to-date knowledge of effectiveness, safety and cost of medications that they may prescribe; and possess good communication skills in order to assist individual patients in making informed choices about treatment.

Implied consent

It is sometimes said that the fact that a person comes into hospital means that they are giving consent to anything the consultation deems appropriate. That, however, is not supported in law. There are many choices of available treatment, and when care is provided, there must be evidence that the patient has agreed to that particular course. Similarly, it is said that when an unconscious patient is treated in an A+E department, he implies consent to be treated. This, however, is likewise not so. An unconscious patient implies nothing. The professional care for him or her in the absence of consent is part of their duty of care for the patient out of necessity in an emergency and could defend any subsequent action for trespass to the person on that basis. This would now be acting under the statutory duty provided by the Mental Capacity Act to act in the best interests of a mentally incapacitated person.

The weakness of implied consent is, however, that it is not always clear that the patient is agreeing to what the nurse intends to do. Thus, the patient who rolls up his or her sleeve for blood pressure to be taken would get a shock when blood is taken or an injection given. To avoid such misunderstandings, it is preferable if the nurse/healthcare professional tells the patient what is to happen and obtains a spoken consent.

Record keeping

The sharing of accurate information between multidisciplinary team members is vitally important. It is highlighted by the Crown Report (DH, 1989) that good record communication between healthcare professionals and patients, and between different professionals, is essential for high quality healthcare.

Good record keeping in relation to prescribing is essential and provides an efficient method of communication and dissemination of information between members of the multidisciplinary team. The healthcare record is a tool for communication within the team. It should provide clear evidence of the care planned, the decisions made, the care delivered and the information shared.

The prescribing details, together with other details of the consultation with the patient, should be entered into the patient's record. The record should clearly indicate the date, the amount of the items prescribed and the quantity prescribed (dose, frequency and treatment duration) at the time of generating the prescription. Where nurses hold separate nursing records, they have the responsibility to ensure this information is entered into the medical records as soon as possible and preferably contemporaneously. All health professionals qualified to prescribe should have access to the relevant patient records. Ideally, these records should be shared between team members.

Self-assessment test

1 Name the four areas of accountability as a non-medical prescriber.
2 How do you ensure that you work within your scope of practice?
3 What is vicarious liability and why is it important?
4 What is the legislation related to non-medical prescribing?

5 Which healthcare professionals can prescribe independently?
6 What are the additional requirements when prescribing controlled drugs?
7 What is the definition of duty of care?

Reflective exercise

You have now read through and studied the contents of this chapter, and it is time for you to reflect on what you have learnt and consider how you are going to relate this to your prescribing practice. From what you have learnt, consider how this will influence what you prescribe. Will the information that you have learnt change any of the prescribing decisions that you thought you may have had previously, and if so, what, how and why?

References

Avery, G. (2013). *Law and ethics in nursing and healthcare. An introduction.* London: Sage Publications.

Bartlett, E., & Eaton, G. (2019). Clinical negligence. In: G. Eaton, ed. *Law and ethics for paramedics, an essential guide.* Bridgwater: Class Professional Publishing, pp. 107–122.

Beauchamp, T.L., & Childress, J.F. (2013). *Principles of biomedical ethics* (7th ed.). Oxford: Oxford University Press.

Brack, G. (2014). Nurse prescribing and vicarious liability. *Nurse Prescribing.* 12(3), 147–149.

Chartered Society of Physiotherapy. (2018). *Practice guidance for physiotherapist supplementary and/or independent prescribers* (4th ed.). Available at https://www.csp.org.uk/publications/practice-guidance-physiotherapist-supplementary-andor-independent-prescribers-safe-use. Accessed 28 April 2020.

College of Paramedics. (2018). Practice guidance for paramedic independent and supplementary prescribers. Available at https://collegeofparamedics.co.uk/COP/Professional_development/Medicines_and_Independent_Prescribing/COP/ProfessionalDevelopment/Medicines_and_Independent_Prescribing.aspx?hkey=04486919-f7b8-47bd-8d84-47bfc11d821a. Accessed 28 April 2020.

Crown Prosecution Service. (2019). Gross negligence manslaughter. Available at https://www.cps.gov.uk/legal-guidance/gross-negligence-manslaughter. Accessed 13 April 2020.

Davey, P., Rathmell, A., Dunn, M., Foster, C., & Salisbury, H. (2017). *Medical ethics, law and communication*. Chichester: John Wiley and Sons Ltd.

Department of Health (DH). (1989). Report on the advisory group on nurse prescribing (Crown Report). London, DH.

Department of Health. (2009). Reference guide to consent for examination or treatment (2nd ed.). Available at https://assets.publishing.service.gov.uk/government/uploads/system/uploads/attachment_data/file/138296/dh_103653__1_.pdf. Accessed 28 April 2020.

Dimond, B. (2011). *Legal aspects of medicines* (2nd ed.). London: Quay Books Division.

Griffith, R., & Dowie, I. (2019). *Dimond's legal aspects of nursing. A definitive guide to law for nurses* (8th ed.). Harlow: Pearson Education Ltd.

Health and Care Professions Council. (2016). Standards of conduct, performance and ethics. Available at https://www.hcpc-uk.org/standards/-standards-of-conduct-performance-and-ethics/. Accessed 30 April 2020.

Health and Care Professions Council. (2019). Standards for prescribing. Available at https://www.hcpc-uk.org/standards/standards-relevant-to-education-and-training/standards-for-prescribing/. Accessed 30 April 2020.

Johnston, C., & Bradbury, P. (2016). *100 cases in clinical ethics and law* (2nd ed.). Florida: CRC Press.

National Institute for Health and Care Excellence. (2020a). Prescription writing. Available at https://bnf.nice.org.uk/guidance/prescription-writing.html. Accessed 30 April 2020.

National Institute for Health and Care Excellence. (2020b). Controlled drugs and drug dependence. Available at https://bnf.nice.org.uk/guidance/controlled-drugs-and-drug-dependence.html. Accessed 30 April 2020.

Nursing and Midwifery Council. (2018a). The code. Professional standards of practice and behaviour for nurses, midwives and nursing associates. Available at https://www.nmc.org.uk/standards/code/. Accessed 28 April 2020.

Nursing and Midwifery Council. (2018b). Part 3: Standards for prescribing programmes. Available at https://www.nmc.org.uk/globalassets/sitedocuments/education-standards/programme-standards-prescribing.pdf. Accessed 28 April 2020.

Royal Pharmaceutical Society. (2016). A competency framework for all prescribers. Available at https://www.rpharms.com/resources/frameworks/-prescribers-competency-framework. Accessed 28 April 2020.

Williams, N. (2018). Gross negligence manslaughter in healthcare. The report of a rapid policy review. Available at https://assets.publishing.

service.gov.uk/government/uploads/system/uploads/attachment_
data/file/717946/Williams_Report.pdf. Accessed 28 April 2020.

Legislation

Children Act 1989
Human Medicines Regulations 2012
Medicines Act 1968
Mental Capacity Act 2005
Misuse of Drugs Act 1971
Misuse of Drugs Regulations 2001.

Legal Cases

Bawa-Garba v GMC [2018]
Bolam v Friern Hospital Management Committee [1957]
Bolitho v City and Hackney Health Authority [1998]
Donoghue v Stevenson [1932]
Gillick v West Norfolk and Wisbech Area Health Authority [1985]
R v Adomako [1994]
R v Bawa-Garba [2015]

6 Psychological influences and issues of concordance

Alison Pooler

Introduction

Deciding on what to prescribe and writing a prescription is a complex situation you will face when you take on a prescribing role, as there are many influences that will be evident on your prescribing practice and many outcomes, which may not always prove positive. Consideration of the different influences and factors upon your prescribing practice needs to be made for you to develop into a safe and effective prescriber.

This chapter covers the psychological and sociological models and influences on the prescribing of medications and the consultation and decision-making process, why health care professionals prescribe and why patients want prescriptions and what other influencing factors there are in this prescribing relationship, including those from the multidisciplinary team.

Learning objectives

By the end of this chapter, you should be able to

- Understand the principles and theories behind what and why patients have different beliefs of their conditions and illnesses and how this affects the prescribing partnership.
- Discuss why healthcare professionals prescribe and the influences on this process.
- Discuss why patients want prescriptions and the influences on them.

The patient's health beliefs

Stewart and Roter (1989) discuss in their "disease–illness model" an analysis of the different perspectives of patient and practitioner for the sickness they are experiencing. According to this model, disease is the cause of sickness in terms of its pathophysiology, whilst illness is the patient's unique experience of sickness. One can exist without the other; for example, someone can have a disease but no symptoms (e.g. hypertension) and have symptoms but no disease (e.g. travel sickness).

Diseases may cause a widely varying illness experience in different individuals, due to their concerns, expectations, support systems and previous experiences (Silverman et al., 1998). Patient's illness experience depends, to a great extent, upon their perspective on their health. Rotter's locus of control (LOC) theory and Rosenstock's health belief model (HBM; Ogden, 2004) go some way to explaining why patients have such widely varying health experiences.

LOC is concerned with the extent to which an individual feels able to influence and control their own life. According to the LOC theory, people's health beliefs fall into three broad categories:

- **Internal LOC:** People with an internal LOC tend to believe that they are responsible for their own health and that what happens to them is the result of their own actions. They tend to prefer explanations and discussion and will want to be involved in decision-making about their health.
- **External LOC:** People with an external LOC tend to have a fatalistic attitude to life and health and will be reluctant to make any exchanges as they believe that their future is mapped out and there is nothing they can do to alter it.
- **Powerful others:** People tend to see the responsibility for their health as lying with other people, such as health professionals. They will be reluctant to take responsibility for their own health and are most happy with an authoritarian approach.

Obviously, these are the broad categories and most people lie somewhere along the continuum. They may adopt a different belief system for different situations they are in. An awareness of a person's LOC can help the practitioner to adopt the most appropriate skills in consultation, decision-making and the ultimate prescribing decision.

The HBM (Ogden, 2004) suggests that individuals' motivation to take any health-related action is dependent upon four factors:

- **Perceived vulnerability:** Those who believe that they are likely to develop lung cancer are more likely to seek advice to help them stop smoking.
- **Perceived seriousness:** Hypertension may not be regarded as a serious condition to some people as it does not cause them any symptoms or feel unwell. To others who have had a relative die from a stroke or heart attack, their perception of having hypertension will be different and they are more likely to comply with treatment and advice given to them.
- **Perceived benefits:** People weigh up the advantages and disadvantages of a particular course of action. To the individual with high blood pressure, the side effects of the medication may outweigh any supposed benefit.
- **Perceived barriers:** The various barriers a person would need to overcome to go along with the suggested course of action, including physical, psychological and financial. To the person unconvinced of the need to treat high blood pressure, the financial implications of the prescription charges may prove to be the final disincentive.

This is a very basic overview of the HBM, as there are other factors such as previous experience, influence of peers and the media, which all play a part in the person's perceptions of the situation. It is recommended that you read about this model in more depth and this can be found in the *Health Psychology* book by Jane Ogden, at the end of this chapter or in any other health psychology book.

An awareness of these factors may help the practitioner to understand the patient's particular anxieties and to tailor their interviews accordingly, especially when concordance with the prescribed medication is desired.

Effective patient interviewing and history taking

The goal of an effective interview, in the context of prescribing, is to gather enough relevant information to form a database of information for the presenting episode and prescribe the appropriate medication.

Eliciting is a key skill within interviewing and one that requires practice in order to use it to its full potential. Asking questions and getting the required information are different things and can require different approaches. Giving the patient the opportunity to express their concerns is therefore key. Evidence suggests that patients often have more than one problem and that the severity of the problem, to them, is not linked to the order in which they disclose it.

Evidence from a study by Beckman and Frankel (1984) found that in only 23% of consultations was the patient allowed to complete their opening statement of concerns. Furthermore, of the 52 patients in the study, only 1 managed to complete their whole story of their complaint. The average interruption took place after 18 seconds.

When consultations are time restricted, there can be a temptation to concentrate on objective health data and gathering of facts at the expense of more subjective information, yet it is this that will tell you how the presenting problem is affecting the patient's daily living and is therefore highly significant. Within a holistic assessment, it is important that both types of data are treated with equal importance.

For patients, disclosing information about a physical set of symptoms may be easier and therefore introduced earlier in the conversation. This illustrates why allowing the patient to explain their concern fully is important. Subjective health data can also only be verified by the patient and as such may influence any prescribing decisions by the health professional/prescriber and provide an indication of likely concordance.

Whatever data you collect, your approach should be systematic and logical. The use of a simple mnemonic framework can help in focusing open and closed questioning, providing a basis on which to use eliciting skills to gain the information you need. There are many in current use in healthcare, an example of which is SWIPE.

When did it Start?

What makes it Worse?

What causes Improvement?

Is there a Pattern?

What is the Evaluation? (What is being done to make it better?)

Another example is TROCARSSS (Time, Rapidity, Occurrence, Characteristics, Associations, Relief, Site, Spread, Severity).

What if any; do you use in your own clinical area. Provide some information for discussion within the class.

Decision-making for safe prescribing

Decision-making is the portion of the consultation in which the synthesis of all information takes place and the prescribing decision is primarily made. It is a combination of clinical/diagnostic reasoning and hypothesis formation. Historically, this aspect of care has been within the medical domain, but with the expansion of professional roles, such as prescribing for nurses and allied health professions (AHPs), this aspect of care is more wide spread.

In order to be successful in making a diagnosis, the patient must interpret information gained from the patient, clinical signs and symptoms and relate these to the following three areas of knowledge and skills:

1 Evidence-based knowledge gained from professional training
2 Current and past clinical experience
3 Clinical knowledge and performance of techniques

These three elements, combined with the patient's history, make up the foundation on which to base clinical/diagnostic reasoning.

Diagnostic reasoning may be understood as a hypothetic-deductive reasoning approach. In this approach, an initial hypothesis (not a diagnosis) is made based on initial presentation and patient-led information, coupled with the information from diagnostic tests and physical examination. Diagnostic reasoning allows for differentiate diagnosis; the combination of symptoms described by the patient, signs, laboratory data, illness profiles, knowledge of demographics and social influences that added together gives the widest scope on which to reach a conclusion.

Having gathered the information and detected the cues, deciding what to do with this information becomes the central skill within the consultation. Without this, it is not possible to make a sound prescribing decision. Algorithms and IT software have been developed to improve decision-making, but the important aspect here is to remember that they are just there to support your decisions, not a substitute for the development of key clinical and cognitive skills.

Dysfunctional consultations

Consultations can close in a manner that is unsatisfactory to the patient or professional, or both. These consultations can be said to be dysfunctional. Much of the study of dysfunctional consultations comes from medicine. However, the reasons cited have relevance to prescribing by non-medical professionals.

A consultation can be said to be dysfunctional from the patient's perspective if

1   The objectives of the patient are not met or are altered.
2   The patient feels the initial complaint is being trivialised.

This has links to both health-seeking behaviour and health LOC. The individual questions whether their health is under their own control or that of others.

Goffman (1990) suggests that people give others that kind of impression that will lead them to act voluntarily in accordance with their objectives. Therefore, not all self-presentations are positive. In some cases, the impressions people try to convey are far from desirable, such as in pursuit of medication that is not needed.

A consultation can be said to be dysfunctional from the professional perspective if

1   The objectives of the professional are not met or are altered.
2   The professional recommends a course of action that the patient refuses.
3   The patient gives a less effective treatment for the sake of maximising concordance, but feels frustrated that their recommendations are rejected.

For both patients and professionals, satisfaction, compliance and concordance can be considered indicators of dysfunction. Marinker (1998) suggests that only about 50% of patients with chronic disease take their medication as prescribed. With the traditional model of compliance, the patient brings a problem to the professional, who recommends a treatment based on evidence of the disease, and the patient's beliefs and values are seen to distract from the science of treatment and cure.

Within concordance, dysfunction can be minimised by patient and professional who, though holding differing standpoints, form a therapeutic alliance. This is confirmed by Stewart et al. (1979) who found a positive relationship between professional and patient, and a patient-centred approach is the most likely to ensure concordance. In relation to general practice, Larson and Lars (1991) found that failure to explore the patient's expectations of the consultation, the patient's perception of their presenting health problem, information about the advice given to the patient and the relevance of the advice given to the patient.

Byrne and Long (1989) highlight the following as contributors to dysfunctional consultations and the resultant non-concordance with prescribed medication:

1   Rejecting patients offers (we'll talk about that next time)
2   Reinforcing self-position (this will be the best for you)
3   Denying the patient (that is not relevant)
4   Refusing the patients ideas (that will not help your condition)
5   Not paying attention and doing something else
6   Evading questions and changing the subject
7   Not responding to feelings
8   Taking over or interrupting the patient

All of the above needs to be avoided if you are to make a sound and safe prescribing decision and a resultant prescription for medication.

Why prescribe?

Why do we prescribe medicines? Why do patients want prescriptions for medicines? The answer is concerned with the biomedical model, where the patient presents with an illness and the prescriber tries to provide the means to help the patient. This is only a small part of the prescribing relationship, because in reality, prescribing is a more complex social interaction. Unless we understand this, and understand why prescribers and patient behave as they do, we cannot understand prescribing.

Sociological models

There are a number of medical sociological models or theories that have been developed, which can help to explain prescribing behaviour:

1 Lay belief system
2 Legitimisation and sanctioning
3 The sick role
4 Medicalisation

Why do we prescribe?

The obvious answer would be due to a desire to use the pharmacological effect of a drug to improve the patient's condition. Harris et al. (1990) describe this as the respectable answer, but also found that doctors often prescribe even when they anticipate no real medical benefit from the drug. They identified a number of non-biomedical reasons for prescribing medications.

- To avoid doing something else, e.g. referring the patient to hospital or another service
- To maintain contact, e.g. by not annoying the patient by refusing to prescribe an antibiotic so that the patient remains on their list. This is very common in long-term conditions
- To temporise and gain time: Often the diagnosis is not clear in early disease, so prescribing may allow time for the disease process to become clear or if it is a self-limiting disease. This temporising is also part of the first two points above, e.g. to avoid referring unnecessarily. It may also be important to allow patients time to understand their own disease or condition.

- To satisfy the urge to give: There may be a very human feeling that something has to be given to the patient out of compassion, even if what is given is inappropriate, e.g. prescribing calpol for a mother with three children so she doesn't have to pay for it over the counter.
- To terminate the consultation
- To maintain the professional role
- To use the power of the placebo effect
- To legitimise the patient's illness
- To earn money in pharmaceutical industry sponsored post marketing surveillance studies
- To avoid medico legal fears
- To avoid being called out on an emergency visit, e.g. Friday afternoon prescribing of antibiotics
- Habit or previous experience

Is prescribing for these non-medical reasons or allowing your decision to prescribe being influenced by any of these rational? From a strict biomedical standpoint it may be not, but from many other viewpoints it may be. There is a balance to be struck and many considerations to be made on an individual basis.

Other influences on prescribing

- **Colleagues:** Senior colleagues (opinion leaders) are very influential in encouraging the issuing of a prescription or not in particular circumstances. Peer pressure is a very important factor, as most of us do not like to be too out of line with everyone else. This factor is often used by pharmaceutical companies or health authorities to influence prescribing.
- **Pharmaceutical companies:** They can be very influential, in both a positive and a negative way. They can be a very valuable source of education, but it has to be remembered that their role is to make profits by encouraging more use of their products. Good advice on how to manage pharmaceutical representatives was provided by the Drugs and Therapeutics Bulletin (Anon, 1983) – see reference at the end of this chapter.

- **The National Health Service (NHS):** Efforts by the NHS to influence our prescribing are particularly powerful psychological and social influences on us to prescribe in certain ways. There are prescribing budgets to remind us of the costs of what we prescribe, which are set by the trusts. This is also linked with clinical governance of the care provided, including prescribing. We are constantly being pushed to improve the quality of prescribing while containing costs as much as possible. This is done in various ways such as the following:

  a Professionally by education
  b Newsletters
  c Peer support or pressure
  d Managerially by budget setting
  e Configuring services, e.g. how many nurse independent or AHP supplementary prescribers are needed and where

- **Placebo:** comes from the Latin phrase "I will please", and is an inert or inactive substance knowingly prescribe for its non-specific psychological or psycho-physiological therapeutic effect. The development of the randomised controlled trial showed the true power of the placebo effect. For example, in mild depression, the response to a supposedly therapeutic drug might be 70%, but the response to a placebo in the same trial can be as high as 60%. This reflects in part the national history of the condition, that is, most patients get better whatever you do, but also the ability of a placebo to bring about a physical improvement by influencing the patients beliefs and expectations.

Some feel that the use of placebos is unethical, but it is also recognised the important effects of reassurance to the patient which is brought about by the use of placebos. It, however, should be used with caution and as rarely as possible.

Why do patients want prescriptions? Or do they really want prescriptions?

It is suggested that prescribers tend to overrate the patients' expectation of a prescription. Indeed the public are often adverse to wanting certain drugs and often seek alternatives. Some people will refuse prescriptions, either directly or indirectly, by simply not getting the prescription filled or not taking the tablets.

Reasons for wanting a prescription include the following:

a   The patient perceives therapeutic effect for themselves or others, which is almost a biomedical type of belief in the power of medicines. However, this may not be in line with the professionals' more scientific beliefs on this. There are also sometimes elements of superstition around the power of the prescription, and this can be linked back to the HBM discussed earlier.

b   To avoid expenditure, that is, getting a prescription for calpol rather than buying it over the counter.

c   To sanction or make contact with the doctor, nurse or AHP

d   To achieve recognition of the sick role and to legitimise time off work or school

e   Suggestion by an opinion leader, e.g. parent, colleague, friend, etc.

f   Requirement of a repeat of a previous experience, e.g. having a sore throat and getting a prescription for antibiotics previously, will want them again this time

g   To receive a gift; as many people take drugs they may not of really wanted or needed because they didn't want to reject the advice given

Patients and the media

Increasingly the media influences us all in our day-to-day lives and habit, including the medicines we take or desire. It portrays sensation and tends to see medicines as either wonder drugs or killer drugs. In recent years, the media coverage of some new drugs has been intense, for instance Viagra and Herceptin. This has certainly raised public awareness of the drug, which may be good if it allows some patients with conditions which can be helped by the drugs. It can also be dangerous in allowing patients to misunderstand the drugs and believe they are suitable for them to take. There, however, has been little media coverage about the side effect of such drugs and the suitability of the drugs for certain groups of patients.

Another example is the uptake of measles mumps and rubella (MMR) vaccination, which fell drastically after adverse publicity that it might be linked with autism or inflammatory bowel disease. Statements by various scientific bodies have not been able to redress the powerful negative perceptions in some parts of the general public, and as a result, there is now a real risk of an epidemic of these possibly serious childhood illnesses.

There is a dilemma here; the professional might like the public's access to such information restricted since it might actually harm the patients; on the other hand, it might benefit patients who are not receiving medications they should or who can learn more about the medicines they are taking. The key concern here should be access to unbiased information which we should encourage, but which is sadly not often available.

Self-assessment test

1 Explain the three broad categories of the LOC model.
2 Name the four factors that affect patients' motivation to take health-related actions, according to the HBM.
3 Name two simple mnemonic frameworks for interviewing and history taking.
4 Name five contributing factors to dysfunctional consultations.
5 Name four sociological theories/models developed to explain prescribing behaviour.
6 Identify five non-biomedical reasons why healthcare professionals prescribe.
7 Name five reasons why patients want a prescription.

Reflective exercise

You have now read through and studied the contents of this chapter, and it is time for you to reflect on what you have learnt and how you are going to relate this to your prescribing practice. From what you have learnt, consider how this this will influence what you prescribe. Will the information that you have learnt change any of the prescribing decisions that you thought you may have had previously, and if so, what, how and why?

References

Anon. (1983). Getting good value from drug representatives. *Drug and Therapeutic Bulletin.* 21(4), 13–15.

Byrne, P., & Long, B. (1989). *Doctors talking to patients.* London: RCGP.

Goffman, E. (1990). *The preservation of self in everyday life.* Harmondsworth: Penguin.

Harris, C.M., Heywood, P.L., & Claydon, A.D. (1990). *The analysis of prescribing in general practice; a guide to audit and research.* London: HMSO.

Larson, C.H.R., & Lars, L. (1991). Connections between the quality of consultations and patient compliance in general practice. *Family Practice.* 8(2), 154–160.

Marinker, M. (1998). Compliance is not all. *British Medical Journal.* 316(-7125), 151.

Ogden, J. (2004). *Health Psychology, a textbook* (3rd ed.). Berkshire: Open University Press.

Paiguana, H. (1997). Consultations; in practice. *Practice Nursing.* 8(8), 20–22.

Silverman, J., Kurtz, S., & Draper, J (1998). *Skills for communicating with patients.* Oxon: Radcliffe Medical Press.

Stewart, M.A., & Roter, D. (1989). *Communicating with medical patients.* Newbury Park: Sage Publications.

Stewart, M.A., McWhinney, I.R., & Buch, C.W. (1979). The client/patient relationship and its effect on outcome. *Journal of the Royal College of General Practitioners.* 29, 77–82.

7 The public health context of prescribing

Alison Pooler

Introduction

This chapter examines the meaning of public health and the public health dimension of prescribing. The three main areas of discussion are antimicrobial resistance, use and misuse of drugs and iatrogenesis. The public health philosophy if prescribing helps to maintain a focus on the true determinants of health, serves justice in healthcare and promotes a holistic approach to practice.

Learning objectives

By the end of this chapter, students should be able to

- Discuss the basic principles of public health.
- Understand the concept of antimicrobial resistance and how this may relate to the antimicrobials own prescribing practice.
- Understand the concept of drug misuse and abuse and how this may impact on their own prescribing practice.
- Discuss and analyse the concept of iatrogenesis and relate the ways of preventing this to their own prescribing practice.
- Be able to relate to the importance of organisations such as the Committee for Safe Medicines (CSM) and the Medicines and Healthcare Products Regulatory Agency (MHRA) and the relevance of their work to their own prescribing practice.

The principles of public health

Public health is concerned with the ability of the many to live healthily and any intervention aimed at sustaining or improving this. This is governed by universal principles of community collaboration, empowerment and health as a human right. Public health has been the concern of civilisation since ancient times, but the huge shifts in population that accompanied the industrialisation and urbanisation of Victorian Britain and the resultant increase in squalor poverty and disease created a backdrop for major humanitarian campaigns in favour of prison reform, sanitary regulation, effective systems for sewage and waste disposal, the provision of basic clean housing and education regarding hygiene and nutrition. It was also during this time that limits began to be set on working hours and conditions not least those pertaining to children (Naidoo & Wills, 2005).

The public health reforms of the nineteenth and twentieth centuries, together with better healthcare, have led to an improved level of health for all, which is observable in average life expectancy increases from 45.5 years in men and 49 years in women in 1901, to 76 years in men and 81 years in women in 2000. However, the infectious disease epidemics linked to former prevailing social conditions have been replaced by a new breed of conditions such as cardiovascular disease, cancer, diabetes, acquired immunodeficiency disease (AIDS) and mental illness (Colgrove, 2002). All these conditions have the potential to outstrip the capacity to treat them (DOH, 2004).

The increase in mobility of populations across the world, whether for reasons of economic migration, trade and commerce or political asylum, has led to a greater multicultural mix in most nations and with it a more complex variety of health needs. The economic world recession of the latter part of the twentieth century left many communities in need of investment and regeneration. Relative poverty and social exclusion have resulted in low social morale and fragmented neighbourhood networks. The advent of the 24/7 society has brought with it changing patterns of working and living, which do not sit well with an inflexible primary health care provision confined to office hours.

Increasingly sedentary routines, widespread use of labour-saving technology and the reduction of time and space reserved for sport as part of the school curricula mean that physical exercise no longer assumes a natural place at the heart of individual lifestyles. Dietary habits have changed so that a greater proportion is occupied by foods with a high glycaemic index as well as saturated and hydrogenated fats (Ebelling et al., 2002). Fast and convenience foods, in company with potentially misleading information about their content, have exacerbated this trend. These factors have been blamed for increased levels of obesity and cardiovascular disease (Baltas et al., 2000; Dietz, 2001).

Prolonged life expectancy has brought with it an increase in chronic illnesses and greater caring responsibilities for a shrinking younger population. A larger ageing population and the unprecedented number of immunosuppressed patients due to surgery or treatment for conditions such as cancer would not have survived in the past, and this means the population is more vulnerable to disease, which all has an impact on the prescription of medicines.

Antimicrobial resistance

This is a collective term referring to the changes that take place in microbes that serve to protect them by reducing or negating the effectiveness of therapeutic agents designed to fight infection. Antimicrobials have stood at the forefront of medical treatment and biomedical scientific advancement for almost three quarters of a century. The discussion point is the problems this has now created. Resistance to penicillin was observed as early as 1940. Now the ability of microbes to develop a variety of mechanisms that sustain them in the face of the most powerful antimicrobial agents poses one of the biggest threats to public health in the twenty-first century. Consequently, major infectious diseases have become more difficult to treat, and the scale and imminence of the presenting danger should not be underestimated.

Antibiotic consumption has risen by 6.5% over the past four years in England, and increased antibiotic prescribing is fuelling increased resistance in bacteria (PHE, 2018). Estimates suggest that as many as half of all patients who visit their general practitioners

(GP) with a cough or cold leave with a prescription for antibiotics. One in three individuals still believes that antibiotics will treat coughs and colds, and one in five expects antibiotics when they visit their GP (PHE, 2018). Seventy-four per cent of all antibiotic prescriptions are generated in Gp surgeries as this is the first point of contact for people seeking medical help.

We cannot afford to lose the power of antibiotics, as they are a vital tool for modern medicine and not just for the treatment of infections. We also need them to avoid infections during chemotherapy, caesarean sections and other surgery. Unless action is taken to address the problem of antibiotic resistance, routine operations could become deadly in just 20 years' time, as healthcare professionals lose the ability to treat infections. A failure to address the problem of antibiotic resistance could result in an estimated 10 million deaths per year globally by 2050, at a cost of £66 trillion to the global economy.

Routes of resistance

Pharmacodynamic variety in antimicrobials means that bacteria have the capacity to develop and retain multiple resistances. Resistance has been spread by spontaneous mutations, by transposons and by exchange of DNA materials via plasmids. In spontaneous mutations, a mutant gene imports resistance to a microbe, which then thrives and divides. Transposons are sections of DNA that can replicate themselves and code for resistance. Each section has end segments at either end that, aided by the enzyme transposase, migrate to other parts of the microbes genomes and insert themselves there, rather like "cut and pasting" in an electronic document This migration has led to transposons being informally labelled jumping genes.

Plasmids are circular packets of genetic material that often exists close to the bacterial cell wall ad that codes for replication of resistance, which can be unilaterally transferred during conjugation with other bacteria. Transposons use plasmids as stepping stones. Resistant DNA can also be absorbed by the bacterium from the external environment.

Although this is a very simplified summary of how resistance develops at a cellular level, it illustrates the complexities which occur and how we should think carefully before prescribing an antibiotic for no valid reason.

Contributory factors to antimicrobial resistance

There is no one solitary causative factor at the root of this situation. Many features of our modern world that at a glance may appear unrelated have contributed to the rise in resistant microbes. It is likely, however, that these factors fall into one or more of the following categories:

- Mobility among individuals, communities and groups
- Herded populations
- Suboptimum prescribing practice
- Poor adherence to prescribed regimens
- Suboptimal standards of infection control
- Other misuse of antimicrobials

The Health Protection Agency (HPA) requires all microbiology centres to monitor and report resistance trends. In turn, it collates these statistics to produce a national picture and make recommendations as to good proactive prescribing practice and infection control through evidenced-based guidelines.

Evidence-based prescribing of antimicrobials includes short, three-day courses, matched with penetration times for conditions such as uncomplicated cystitis or otitis media. Non-prescribing behaviour, refraining from unnecessary treatment with antimicrobials, is equally important.

Tackling inappropriate antibiotic prescribing

Improving prescribing practice can be difficult, especially in the face of patient demands. But evidence suggests that informing prescribers of their prescribing patterns compared with peer professionals can help. National guidance on antimicrobial stewardship has been published by the National Institute for Health and Care Excellence (NICE), which recommends benchmarking individual prescribing rates against local and national rates and trends.

Public Health England (PHE) has developed two national toolkits to improve antibiotic prescribing in England: TARGET (Treat Antibiotics Responsibly, Guidance, Education, Tools) and Start Smart. It also has developed a quality premium payment for antibiotics use, which incentivises clinical commissioning groups (CCGs) to reduce prescribing of antibiotics by at least 1% from 2013 to 2014 levels year on year (PHE, 2015).

Drug misuse and abuse

Substance abuse or the use of drugs for non-therapeutic and recreational purposes has been present in developed and underdeveloped countries for hundreds of years. It has now reached epidemic proportions and lies at the root of many of the dysfunctional features of society such as crime. The abuse of major toxic substances has been linked to cardiovascular disease, hepatitis C, the induction of mental illness, HIV/AIDS and premature death (Fergusson et al., 2005; Patrick et al., 2001; Weaver et al., 2003). Drugs and substances abused include the following:

- Alcohol
- Tobacco
- Opiate derivatives, e.g. kaolin morphine and codeine linctus
- Methylphenidate (Ritalin) is used for treatment of ADHD, but if abused it is crushed and injected or inhaled. It is also an appetite depressant so it is abused by people trying to lose weight. It is known as kiddie coke or vitamin R on the street
- Drug cocktails such as benzodiazepines and anxiolytics with alcohol
- Anabolic steroids
- Laxatives
- Ecstasy
- Ketamine (angel dust, special K or Kit Kat)
- Crack cocaine and a range of street drugs which are evolving on our streets such as monkey dust

There are many long-term diseases such as mental health illnesses, and pulmonary and cardiovascular diseases that people abusing such drugs succumb to. There is also the issue of safe prescribing for these people, because of altered pharmacokinetics and pharmacodynamics that may occur because of the abuse of these drugs and the interactions that may occur with legitimate prescribed drugs and medicines. Advice should be sought for the appropriateness and safety of prescribing drugs for these individuals.

Preventing iatrogenesis

Iatrogenesis as it relates to adverse drug reactions is a negative impact on a patient's health status as a result of prescribing, preparation, dispersing and administration of medicines. It has been estimated that drug errors constitute the single largest source of iatrogenic incidents, at 11% (Leape et al., 1995).

Any response to reducing drug errors recognises the complex, fast-paced world in which participants and patients interact. Optimum competency in numeracy alone is sufficient protection against errors in such an environment, in which healthcare professionals are frequently required to multitask.

Drugs that are pre-packed in pharmacies for administration are becoming commonplace, as is the use of the patient's own drugs in formal care settings and drug dispensers that can be used in the patient's own homes.

Good history taking: This is the primary weapon of prevention against adverse drug events. It helps assemble a patient portfolio of past allergies and reactions and present medications; which will include over-the-counter, general sales list, alternate treatments and non-therapeutic as well as prescribed drugs. The more detailed the history, the better the assessment of risk that is facilitated (NPC, 1999). Vulnerable groups such as the elderly, children and those who have multiple disease states or are immunosuppressed deserve special attention (NPC, 1999).

Sharing best practice: Responsibility for CPD, which is shared by health care practitioners and employers, also contributes to drug administration safety (NMC, 2002). The use of significant event audit is now part of established good practice and serves to produce a common team learning process out of an individual error, rather than to apportion blame. Learning that arises out of good practice is also shared. Clinical care pathways and information systems such as Prescribing RatiOnally with Decision support In General practice studY (PRODIGY) (help ensure that evidence-based practice guides and informs prescribing behaviour and provides maps for planning therapeutic intervention (NPC & NPCRDC, 2002).

Reporting unanticipated deviations from the norm: In 2002 the Yellow Card System to report adverse reactions to the CSM and MHRA come into effect. It is the point at which proactive and reactive medicines management occurs, and through the reports generated by the CSM and MHRA, pharmacovigilance and awareness are increased among other prescribers and patient safety benefits accordingly.

Optimum team working: Electronic patient records enhance shared record systems, so that the whole team caring for that patient can see up-to-date records on which to base their clinical and prescribing decisions. The potential for adverse events is therefore reduced, amongst many other positive outcomes.

It is not merely the lack of patient education about prescribed treatment but the lack of sensitivity as to the timeliness of such education, along with failure to genuinely engage the patient's concerns, which results in a breakdown in concordance and consequent adverse drug events and errors (Jacobs, 2002). Educating patients about their medication and treatment, therefore, cannot be merely the depersonalised transfer of information, but like all good teaching is couched in an awareness of the link between meeting leaner needs and assimilation of new knowledge. However, in our efforts to secure safer medicines management, there may still be an even better way forward.

Public health initiatives are always more effective when appropriated by the public and when strengths of leadership and support grounded in the community are harnessed (Laverack, 2005). Practitioners have long recognised that many patients who suffer from chronic disease have through experience developed expertise and skill relating to their conditions that can be shared with others. Formalising this concept of the expert patient, through the development of support and education programmes that are led by service users, has been linked to improved concordance. This is another step towards minimising adverse drug events.

The public health dimension of prescribing

A public health model of prescribing practice does not conform to the traditional biomedical model of care that has until recently dominated the prescribing world. Therapeutic management of cholesterol and obesity in the absence of specific disease states has joined immunisation in the area of primary public health medicine and produced beneficial results. To prescribe in a context of public health is to own a public health philosophy in practice, appreciating the broader health consequences for the individual and the range of treatment options and care packages.

Both prescribing and non-prescribing behaviours should afford an opportunity for patients to explore ways in which they might be enabled to change their life style for the better. This may provide solutions that are alternatives or complementary to a prescription.

In the twenty-first century, a public health approach is required to respond effectively to the challenges to health arising from the patterns of disease associated with the current times. Wherever prescribing takes place, a public health philosophy serves to broaden care beyond the limited boundaries of therapeutic and promotes holistic practice.

Self-assessment test

- What is public health concerned with?
- What universal principles govern public health?
- What does the term "antimicrobial resistance" refer to?
- What three ways has resistance to microbials been spread?
- What are the contributory factors to antimicrobial resistance?
- The abuse of substances has led to many major disease states. Can you name some?
- What is iatrogenesis?
- What is the benefit of the reports produced by the CSM and the MHRA?

Reflective exercise

You have now read through and studied the contents of this chapter, and it is time for you to reflect on what you have learnt and how you are going to relate this to your prescribing practice. From what you have learnt, consider how this will influence what you prescribe. Will the information that you have learnt change any of the prescribing decisions that you thought you may have had previously, and if so, what, how and why?

References

Amaranayake, N., Church, J., Hill, C., Jackson, J., Jackson, J.V., Myers, C., Saeed, Z., Shipsey, C., & Symmonds, T. (2000). *Social trends, 30.* London: HMSO.

Baggott, R. (2000). *Public health, policy and politics* (2nd ed.). Basingstoke: Palgrave MacMillan.

Baltas, G. (2001). Nutritional labelling; issues and policies. *European Journal of Marketing.* 35(5/6), 708–721.

Callaghan, E. (2003). Submit a yellow card to report adverse drug reactions. *Nurse Prescribing Journal.* 1(3), 138–139.

Charalambous, M.P. (2002). Alcohol and the accident and emergency department; a current review. *Alcohol and Alcoholism.* 37(4), 307–312.

Colgrove, J. (2002). The McKeowan thesis; a historical controversy and its enduring influence. *American Journal of Public Health.* 92(5), 725–730.

Curran, H.V., & Morgan, C.A. (2000). Cognitive, dissociative and psychogenic effects of ketamine in recreational users on the night of drug use and 3 days later. *Addiction.* 95(4), 575–590.

Department of Health. (2000). *UK Antimicrobial resistance strategy and action plan.* London: HMSO.

Department of Health. (2004). *Choosing Health, making healthier choices easier.* London: HMSO.

Dietz, W.H. (2001). The obesity epidemic in young children; reduce TV viewing and promote playing. *British Medical Journal.* 322(7282), 313–314.

Downie, G., Hind, C., & Kettle, J. (2000). The abuse and misuse of prescribed and over the counter medicines. *Hospital Pharmacist.* 7(9), 242–250.

Ebelling, C.D., Pawlak, D.B., & Ludwig, D.S. (2002). Childhood obesity; public health crisis, common sense cure. *The Lancet.* 360(9331), 473–482.

Emslie, M.J., & Bond, C.M. (2003). Public knowledge, attitudes and behaviour regarding antibiotics; a survey of patients in general practice. *European Journal of General Practice.* 9(3), 84–90.

Fergusson, D.M., Horwood, L.J., & Ridder, E.M. (2005). Tests of causal linkages between cannabis use and psychiatric symptoms. *Addiction.* 100(3), 354–366.

Health Protection Agency. (2005). *Antimicrobial resistance; inevitable but not unmanageable.* London: HPA.

Jacobs, L. (2002). Are your patients taking what you prescribe? *Permanente Journal.* 6(3), 59–61.

Kutscher, E.C., Lund, B.C., & Perry, P.J. (2002). Anabolic steroids, a review for the clinician. *Sports Medicine.* 32(5), 285–296.

Laverack, G. (2005). *Public Health, power, empowerment and professional practice.* Basingstoke: Palgrave Macmillan.

Leape, L.L., Bates, D.W., Cullen, D.J., Cooper, J., Demonaco, H., Gallivan, T., Hallisey, R., Ives, J., Laird, N., Laffel, G., Nemeskal, R., Peterson, LA., Porter, K., Servi, D., Shea, B.F., Small, S.D., Sweitzer, B.J., Thompson, T., Vliet, M.V. (1995). Systems analysis of adverse drug events. *Journal of the American Medical Association.* 274(1), 35–43.

Naidoo, J., & Wills, J. (2005). *Health promotion, foundations for practice* (2nd ed.). London: Bailliere Tindall.

National Prescribing Centre. (1999). Signposts for prescribing nurses; general principles of good prescribing. *Prescribing Nurse Bulletin.* 1(1), 1–4.

National Prescribing Centre and National Primary Care Research and Development Centre. (2002). *Modernising medicines management, a guide to achieving benefits for patients, professionals and the NHS.* London: NPC.

Nursing Midwifery Council. (2002). *Supporting nurses and midwives through life long learning.* London: NMC.

Patrick, D.M., Tyndall, M.W., Cornelisse, P.G., Lin, K., Sherlock, C.H., Rehart, M.L., Strathdee, S.A., Currie, S.L., Schechter, M.T., & O'Shaughnessy, M.V. (2001). Incidence of hepatitis C virus infection among injection drug users during an outbreak of HIV infection. *Canadian Medical Association Journal.* 165(7), 889–895.

Public Health England. (2018). Health matters; tackling antimicrobial resistance. Available at http://www.gov.uk/government/collections/-health-matters-public-health-issues. Accessed 11 May 2020.

Weaver, T., Madden, P., Charles, V., Stimson, G., Renton, A., Tyrer, P., Barnes, T., Bench, C., Middleton, H., Wright, N., Paterson, S., Shanahan, W., Seivewright, N., & Ford, C. (2003). Co-morbidity of substance misuse and mental illness in community health and substance misuse services. *British Journal of Psychiatry.* 183(4), 304–313.

8 Prescription writing

Alison Pooler

Introduction

This chapter reviews what a prescription is and how it should be completed by the prescriber safely. It also provides information on what the British National Formulary (BNF) is and its content which are an invaluable aid to the prescriber. It also addresses the topic of cost-effective prescribing.

Learning objectives

By the end of this chapter, you should be able to

* Understand the structure and content of the BNF and relate how the different sections of the BNF can be used in clinical practice.
* Understand the principles of cost-effective prescribing and be able to discuss ways that cost-effective prescribing is implemented in your individual clinical area.
* Understand the principle of safe prescribing and how a prescription chart should be completed safely.

What is the BNF and how to use it?

The BNF aims to provide prescribers and their health care professionals with up-to-date information about the use of medicines. It includes key information on the selection, prescribing, dispensing and administration of medicines. All the information in the BNF is drawn from the manufacturers' product license literature, medical and pharmaceutical literature, UK health departments, regulatory authorities and regulatory bodies. Advice comes from clinical literature and reflects, as much as possible, an evaluation from a broad range of sources. It also takes into account national guidelines.

It is design as a rapid reference and includes information on prescribing and dispensing which can be found in the appendices. The main text of the BNF consists of classified information about the drugs available, and this is organised on a systems-based approach, covering all the systems of the body or aspects of care. At the start of every chapter is a section on notes for prescribers, which is important to read as they facilitate the selection of the most suitable treatments. There is also a list of indications, cautions, contraindications, side effect and dose, and then the different preparations are listed along with their prices and dosage packaging. All of this information and the symbols used can be found at the front of the BNF, which we recommend that you read to familiarise yourself with.

Other sections at the front of the BNF include discontinued preparations, new preparations, guidance on prescribing, prescription writing, emergency supply of drugs, controlled drugs and drug dependence, adverse reactions to drugs, prescribing for children, prescribing in palliative care, prescribing for the elderly, prescribing in dental practice, drugs and sport and emergency treatment of poisoning.

There are also appendices at the back of the BNF which include drug interactions, live disease, renal impairment, pregnancy, breast-feeding, intravenous additives, borderline substances, wound management products and elastic hosiery, cautionary and advisory labels for dispensed medicines. You should spend some time to familiarise yourself with the whole of the BNF. Many people just look the drug they want to prescribe up in the index and turn to that particular page, missing out on all this other important and useful information.

Prescription writing

The BNF contains many regulations and guidance notes concerning the writing of prescriptions. The following will deal with the general principles of prescribing.

Practical prescription writing

There are four common types of prescription:

1 Prescriptions in general practice/community (FP10)
2 Hospital prescriptions for in-patients
3 Hospital prescriptions for out-patients
4 Private prescriptions

No matter what type of prescription is being used, there are certain principles which should be followed for all. Principally, a prescription should be a precise, accurate, clear and readable set of instructions. This will ensure the correct drug is given/administered at the correct dose at the right time and to the right patient. The following information must be given on all prescriptions:

- The date the prescription was written
- Identification of the patient by name, age and date of birth. Age should always be given for children under the age of 12 years
- Weight especially in children where many drug dosages are based on weight
- The name of the drug which should preferably be written in capital letters so that it is clear and usually by the generic name, unless a situation requires the brand name to be used
- The dose of the drug for which the following points must be adhered to
- Quantities of 1 gram or more should be written in grams, for example 2 g or 2 grams
- Quantities less than a gram but more than 100 mg should be written in milligrams, for example write 100 mg not 0.1 g
- Quantities less than 1 milligram should be written in micrograms or nanograms, and these units should not be abbreviated as they can lead to confusion and errors, for example 100 micrograms not 0.1 mg, 100 μg, etc.
- If a decimal point cannot be avoided for values less than 1, then place a 0 before it, for example 0.5 mL not .5 Ml

- For liquid medication given orally, the dose should be stated as the number of milligrams in either 5 mL or 10 Ml, since these are readily measured amounts and measuring spoons and cups are given to patients when the medications are dispensed. If the dose of the drug is contained in anything less than 5 ml, the pharmacist usually dilutes it so that it can be given in 5 mL.
- For some drugs a maximum dose should be given, for example for paracetamol, you write 500 mg–1 g every 4–6 hours, do not take more than 4 g in 24 hours.
- Frequency of administration should be clearly stated, for example atenolol 100 mg once daily or amoxicillin 250 mg TDS.

Acceptable and recognised abbreviations may be used which include the following:

OD   – once daily
PRN – as required
BD   – twice a day
TDS – three times a day
QDS – four times a day

Table 8.1 shows a list of common abbreviations that are used when writing prescriptions.

The simpler the instructions of how often to take the drug the better, as this will ensure less prescribing and administration errors occurring on administration. It is also important to explain to the patient what the dosing schedule means in terms of breakfast, lunch, dinner time and bedtime so they fully understand. In hospital the frequency of drug administration is more controlled with the delegation of this being given to health care professionals. In the community, this is not the case and can be confounded by other conditions in the patient which is their ability to remember or understand.

The route and method of administration should be clearly indicated (e.g. oral, intravenous (IV), intramuscular (IM), sublingual), unless it is obvious such as an inhaler or nebuliser, which is stated separately.

Table 8.1 Abbreviations commonly used when writing prescriptions

Abbreviation	Latin meaning	English translation
BD or BID	*Bis in die*	Twice a day
Gutt	*Guttae*	Drops
IM		Intramuscular
IV		Intravenous
NP	*Nomen proprium*	The proper name
OD	*Omni die*	(Once) every day
OM (sometimes written as mane)	*Omni mane*	(once) every morning
ON (sometimes written as nocte)	*Omni nocte*	(once) every night
PO	*Per os*	By mouth
PR	*Per rectum*	By the anal route
PRN	*Pro re nata*	Whenever required
PV	*Per vaginam*	By the vaginal route
QDS/qid	*Quarter die sumendum*	Four times a day
SC		Subcutaneous
STAT	*statim*	Immediately
TDS/tid	*Ter die sumendum*	Three times a day

If you are wanting the drug to be diluted in a solution and given over time, then all of these instructions need to be written down clearly and must include the name and amount of solution and the rate at the which the solution is to be administered especially if being delivered via IV infusion or syringe driver.

The amount of medication to be supplied is important to be clear about. In hospitals the pharmacists organised this depending on the expected length of stay of the patient and the amount to be discharged with from hospital, which is usually a few days' supply so that the patient can then collect a follow-on prescription from their general practitioner (GP). They need this information from the person writing the prescriptions in the ward areas. In the community, the amount to be dispensed has to be stated on the prescription/FP10. This is done by either stating the number of tablets to be supplied for the course of a time period for the treatment or completing the number of days required box at the top of the prescription/FP10.

Instructions on labelling need to be considered, and in the National Health Service (NHS) a drug container will be labelled with the drug name and all the data that the prescriber includes on the prescription. The generic name is usually used and on the FP10s used in the community and GP surgeries there is the instruction NP at the top of the prescription to indicate this. If the prescriber does not want the name of the drug to be written on the label, they must cross out this NP. Generally it is considered more appropriate that the drug name is included on the label. Private prescriptions need to be labelled NP by the prescriber if they want the name of the drug used on the label. An example FP10 is given below.

All prescriptions have to be signed and also include the prescribers' qualifications, for example specialist registrar (SPR) and registered general nurse (RGN). For FP10s the prescriber's address, usually the surgery address, is also completed. For many FP10s, this is pre-printed onto the FP10s when issued or printed on electronic prescription when they are generated. This is so that for any queries regarding the prescription, the pharmacist can contact the prescriber to clarify prior to the drug being dispensed. Private prescriptions are usually written on the prescriber's personal headed note paper or on a specially printed form to avoid any doubt of authenticity.

Repeat prescriptions

Many patients have to take medications long-term so a system for repeat prescriptions is available, which allows for the continuation of a prescription under minimal supervision to ensure continuity of care. In this way, a computerised repeat prescription is generated by a GP surgery receptionist or surgery pharmacist, and the GP or other non-medical prescriber checks it and signs it so the medication can be dispensed. This means the patient doesn't have to be seen every time their prescription runs out, which is more efficient for most conditions. However, there are some where the patient does need to be seen regularly such as the oral contraceptive pill to check blood pressure. Others will have an annual review with possibly blood tests or sooner if any issues occur. About 75% of all items prescribed in the community in the UK are dealt with in this way. However, in order to maintain safety, the following principles must apply:

- The long-term prescription of the drug is justified, and this may require consultation with the patient.
- The duration of each prescription should be no more than three months.
- There should be regular review of all prescriptions annually, and a review date should be set to stop continued repeats after this review date.
- There should be a system which monitors the drugs being dispensed, the frequency of the repeats, any drug interactions and review dates, which all surgeries in the UK have already on their systems (Figure 8.1).

Cost-effective prescribing

Pharmaceutical prescribing represents about 10% of the total NHS budget and is one of the most inflationary elements of spending. The cost of pharmaceuticals is continually rising and the choice of medicines widening. Medicines are one of the most commonly used and important interventions available for health professionals in clinical practice, and their appropriate use can reduce mortality, morbidity and costs falling on other parts of the health service. However, evidence from systematic reviews demonstrates that current prescribing may not always be effective or cost-effective (DH, 2007).

The biggest cost of prescribing comes from primary care, and many government initiatives focus on this area of prescribing. The same principles are used for secondary care though. The Department of health (DH) in their guidance of cost-effective prescribing (DH, 2007) recommend that the following principles should apply:

1   The decision to initiate treatment or change a patient's treatment regime should be based on good quality evidence or guideline, for example from National Institute for Health and Care Excellence (NICE) or other authoritative sources such as the British Thoracic Society.
2   Health professionals should base their prescribing decisions on individual assessments of their patients' clinical circumstances, for example patients whose clinical history suggests they need a particular treatment should continue to receive it.

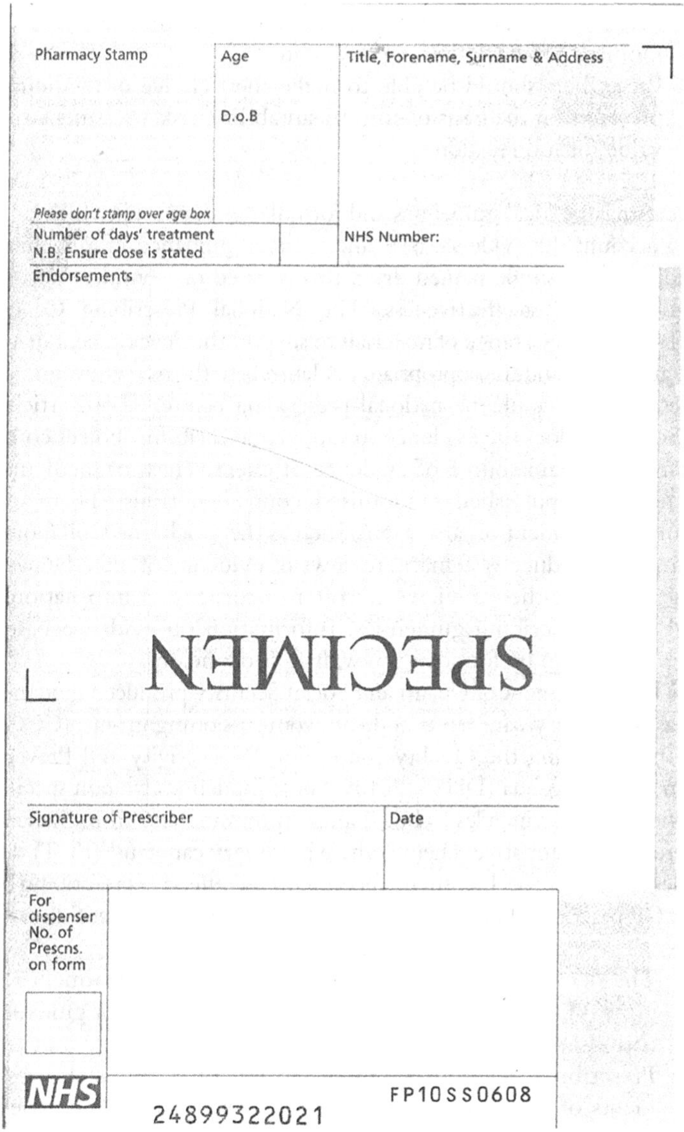

Pharmacy Stamp

Please don't stamp over age box

Age

D.o.B

Title, Forename, Surname & Address

Number of days' treatment
N.B. Ensure dose is stated

NHS Number:

Endorsements

SPECIMEN

Signature of Prescriber

Date

For dispenser
No. of Prescns. on form

NHS

24899322021

FP10SS0608

Figure 8.1 Example of an FP10 prescription chart.

3   The individual patient should be informed about the action
    being taken, and suitable arrangements should be made to
    monitor patient following any switch.
4   Prescribers should be able to make their choice of medicinal
    products on the basis of clinical suitability, risk assessment and
    value for money alone.

There may be local guidelines and formularies drawn up which take into account the evidence base and national guidance. If guidelines recommend a single named drug, this is based on considerations of clinical and cost-effectiveness. The National Prescribing Centre (NPC) provides a range of materials to support the development of local guidelines and the appropriate evidence base (https://www.guidelinesinpractice.co.uk/the-national-prescribing-centre/305502.article).

So where does the evidence to support prescribing choices come from? The main source of evidence of effectiveness of medicines comes from published randomised controlled trials. There are many independent organisations, such as the Cochrane Collaboration, that produce systematic reviews of evidence of effectiveness. The results of these reviews are often incorporated into national and local prescribing guidelines. Information on evidence-based prescribing can be found at www.druginfozone.org.

The Department of Health and Social Security produced guidance to assist primary care trusts and care commissioning groups (CCGs) in implementing the Quality Innovation Productivity and Prevention (QiPP) agenda (DHSS, 2010). These guidelines contain specific advice on the principles to be adopted in framing and administering a prescribing initiative scheme where a primary care trust (PCT) decides to use this mechanism to encourage cost-effective prescribing by the GP practices. The underpinning principles of this are as follows:

–   The decision to initiate treatment or change a treatment regime is based on up-to-date best clinical evidence or guidance (NICE).
–   Prescribing decisions should be based on individual assessments of patients clinical circumstances, for example patient whose clinical history suggests they need a particular treatment should continue to have it.

- Individual patient (or guardian) should be informed about any action being taken and arrangements should be made to involve the patient to ensure they have an opportunity for discussion about their treatment.
- Prescriber should be able to make their choice of medicinal products on the basis of clinical suitability, risk assessment and value for money.
- Medications should be reviewed whenever relevant NICE or alternative guidance is updated if required.

Self-assessment test

1 When writing a prescription for a child under the age of 12 years, what is the legal requirement?
2 On a prescription is it preferable to write 0.5 g or 500 mg? Why?
3 Where can you find information on the evidence base for your prescribing decisions?

Reflective exercise

You have now read through and studied the contents of this chapter, and it is time for you to reflect on what you have learnt and how you are going to relate this to your prescribing practice. From what you have learnt, consider how this will influence what you prescribe. Will the information that you have learnt change any of the prescribing decisions that you thought you may have had previously, and if so, what, how and why?

References

Department of Health. (2007). *Cost effective prescribing principles.* London: HMSO.

Department of Health and Social Services. (2010). *Quality, innovation, productivity and prevention agenda.* London: DHSS.

9 The NMP leads and the multidisciplinary team in prescribing

Alison Pooler and Tracy Hall

Introduction

Every NHS Trust has non-medical prescribing leads (NMP leads). Their role is invaluable in the governance, monitoring, auditing and support of non-medical prescribing staff within their Trust to maintain safety but also ensure continued professional development of these staff. Alongside this effective multidisciplinary team working is paramount to aid the safe prescribing and monitoring of medications for patients.

This chapter outlines some of the responsibilities of the NMP lead role from a community Trust perspective, most of which will be similar to the role within any NHS Trust across the UK. It also covers the concept of multidisciplinary teams working in the arena of non-medical prescribing.

Learning outcomes

After studying this chapter, you will be able to

1 Appreciate the role of the NMP lead within your Trust and how this will link with your own prescribing role.
2 Understand the importance of clinical audit and monitoring of the non-medical prescribing role.
3 Understand the importance of continued professional development once you have qualified as a non-medical prescriber and how the NMP lead is integrated into this.
4 Understand the concept of multidisciplinary teams working and how this relates to non-medical prescribing.

What is multidisciplinary care?

Multidisciplinary care is when professionals from a range of disciplines work together to deliver comprehensive care that addresses as many of the patient's needs as possible. This care can be delivered by a range of professionals functioning as a team under one organisational umbrella or by professionals from a range of organisations across the health sector, to provide a unique team to address that patent's individual needs. As patients' conditions and therefore needs change over time, the composition of the team may also change to reflect this and to ensure adequate care of that patient is maintained for their physical but also psychological needs (Mitchell et al., 2008).

For the team to function effectively, the team needs to work together as effectively and efficiently as possible, and this involves the following:

–   Effective communication
–   Enabling and encouraging supervision
–   Common goals defined

Courage and structures which allow concerns to be raised are as follows:

–   Valuing team members and the matching of roles to ability
–   Mutual respect

The benefits to the health practitioners themselves of effective team working are the development of new skills and approaches, the challenge to traditional norms and values and fostering the appreciation of other roles, the encouragement of innovation and increasing autonomy, and it also allows individuals to focus on specific area of care with the potential to reduce error.

The benefits to the patients include improved access to care, improved patient journey and extended choice of care options. It also helps to co-ordinate services especially for complex problems and reduce hospital admissions and waiting times to receive care requirements (RCN, 2012).

Non-medical prescribing principles and how they relate to Multidisciplinary team (MDT) working

As a non-medical prescriber, your responsibilities are to improve patient care without compromising patient safety and to make it easier and quicker for patients to access medications to aid their recovery or continued maintenance of health. By working effectively in a wider team, you can utilise and draw upon skills of other members of that team, and in the process increase the patient's choice of treatment options and improve the flexibility of health care access for the patient. All of this enhanced team working should improve patient outcomes and be more cost-effective in terms of resources of the health care system. The success of any prescribing depends on the contribution from a number of health care practitioners, some of whom may not be able to prescriber but bring their skills to enable effective team working.

Prescribing in a multidisciplinary team context

For a more streamlined, accessible and flexible service (DH, 2000), patients demand for a high-quality accountable service and for roles which extend beyond traditional boundaries. Acknowledging the range of knowledge and skills held by practitioners and offering them the opportunity to achieve their full potential (DH, 2001, 2002) has meant that the roles of healthcare professionals have changed dramatically over recent years, especially with prescribing roles. These changes have placed a great emphasis on teamwork and multiprofessional cooperation.

The success of non-medical prescribing is dependent upon the contributions from a number of practitioners, including specialist nurses, pharmacists, doctors and other health care professionals, and the ability of these professionals to work together as a team.

In order to work effectively as a team, a number of key elements are required:

i   Effective verbal and written communication
ii   Enabling and encouraging supervisions
iii   Collaboration and common goals

iv Valuing the contributions of team members and matching team roles to ability
v   A culture that encourages team members to seek help
vi Team structure

Underpinning all of these is the need for team members to have a clear understanding of one another's roles, for example the role of the pharmacist will be one that you are asked to discover and spend some time with a pharmacist during the module.

Role of NMP lead

The role of the NMP lead is that primarily of governance and support to colleagues whilst working strategically helping to develop services. A key aspect of the NMP lead role concerns the monitoring of prescribing activity and audit. As an NMP lead, it is their responsibility to ensure that Trust policies, procedures and guidelines are adhered to whilst ensuring that compliance to the local health economy formulary is adhered to wherever possible. In primary care, the local CCGs work alongside the acute hospitals' pharmacy teams to devise a health economy-wide formulary for clinicians to follow; the mental health Trust as specialist providers will lead on the mental health aspect, but as specialists there may be some drugs that only they can prescribe. In a community Trust, the prescribers are commissioned to adhere to 80% formulary compliance, there is an expectation that medics and NMPs will adhere to this as a commissioned service. Patients, however, are not typical and not every item within the formulary would be appropriate to meet their needs; our commissioners expect an 80% compliance rate rather than solely restricted to the formularies requiring 100% compliance. Though there is an expectation that anything prescribed off formulary is exemption reported and a rationale for off-formulary prescribing is stated. The exemption reporting evidence base can be used to influence future formulary changes alongside a formal formulary application to the local new medicines committee led by the pharmacy teams from acute and community providers.

The landscape of the NHS has changed, and services are now often not hosted by the local NHS providers. It is not uncommon for services to be provided by a Trust some miles away placing increased pressures and challenges upon the NMP lead who could be hundreds of miles away from the clinicians they are providing strategic leadership too. Clinicians within these services will also feel frustrated at the difficulties they could encounter when services are transferred across to different care providers, all of whom will have varying governance structures.

For NMP leads, this also brings challenges as they try to support colleagues often hundreds of miles away. It is difficult to engage with clinicians working many miles away and to develop relationships. The ability to be creative and innovative using technology is a requirement of the role when providing support to colleagues within these outreach services.

To be an NMP lead, you have to have had experience as a prescriber and of the pressures being a prescriber brings with it. It is difficult to say no to a demanding patient or where you as a clinician feel that the issue of a prescription is not the appropriate treatment for the clinical presentation you are faced with. The ability to be able to empathise with a colleague faced with the same scenario is beneficial. There is also the requirement to have the strategic overview of the Trust's direction and the subsequent direction of travel when reviewing service provision. The NMP lead in conjunction with senior managers within the Trust is responsible for the identification of areas requiring investment and development of NMPs within commissioned services.

The Trusts' NMP strategies support this vision. NMPs play a vital role in the care provision especially with regard to the vision within the NHS Long-Term Plan (2019); however, as skilled clinicians they are not a substitute for a medic where a medic is required. Overarching medical governance must be met when considering service provision and the development of new services.

Prerequisites of undertaking a non-medical prescribing course are that it must be appropriate for the service the clinician is working within, not just of personal interest to the clinician themselves. Depending upon which qualification is to be studied may also require completion of a physical assessment course beforehand. It is important that the NMP has the underpinning knowledge required to make differential diagnoses and an informed prescribing decision. Therefore, the NMP lead should have knowledge of the clinical area the student NMP works within.

The identification of potential candidates to undertake the NMP course often involves line managers, and the appraisal conversations with the manager will have identified colleagues who wish to acquire these extended skills. The colleague requesting to undertake the NMP course should have had a discussion with the NMP lead prior to starting the application to university process. This discussion will include ascertaining if the potential candidate meets the academic eligibility criteria. Students should have evidence of study at level 6 degree prior to course commencement.

Funding approval from the Trust as well as confirmation of the line manager's support is essential prior to the completion and submission to the university. The line manager is confirming support and release from practice for the designated study hours and that this is a role that will be utilised within their clinical area, whereas the NMP lead confirms that there is also the access to a prescribing budget upon qualification.

Part of the challenges faced by the NMP lead is that of ascertaining the rationale by the clinician who has requested to undertake the course. Unfortunately, Trusts often experience colleagues who do not meet the criteria with it being a service need for increased NMP provision. Often upon completion of the course, some clinicians have either chosen not to use the qualification within practice, or they have chosen to work elsewhere and more recently have left to work within the cosmetic industry. Unfortunately, Trusts are not in a position to be able to request monies back to cover for the NMP course costs from colleagues who either fail to utilise their prescribing within the Trust or leave. As a result of career progression and movement around the country, it would be impossible to determine who would pay money back, especially for colleagues whose partners jobs require them to move around the country such as Trusts adjacent to a military base whereby there are a number of clinicians who are transient as they accompany their partners and families as they change bases. If the NMP lead feels that it is not in the services' interests or that the proposed

NMP applicant does not meet the eligibility criteria, then the application will not be supported. Universities require the support of the NMP lead from Trusts in order to process applications. Practice nurse colleagues should have authorisation from a senior member of their leadership team confirming that upon qualification that they will have access to a prescribing budget.

Whilst the NMP lead is primarily a governance lead role, there is also a pastoral element. It can be quite daunting to physically write a prescription especially if there had been a delay in between undertaking a prescribing course and actually writing a prescription or if roles have changed and there is then the expectation that colleagues will be actively prescribing in the new role. Another component of the role is the ability to be contactable if required. Clinicians may need to ask for advice whether that be reassurance, for instance if it is ok to prescribe paracetamol to an older person residing in a care home knowing the directive from NHS England not to prescribe paracetamol or it could be a complex prescribing question which may need further referral to a pharmacy colleague for a definitive answer. Some colleagues, especially newly qualified, will contact the NMP lead for advice when facing a dilemma.

As an NMP lead, there is the expectation that we will facilitate training sessions, and the professional bodies set the expectation that it is up to individual clinicians to be up to date and responsible for their own learning. As a Trust we will support clinicians and direct them to online resources such as that produced by Health Education England (HEE). HEE produced an online learning resource tool in conjunction with the University of Birmingham known as the SCRIPT Tool. Initially devised for junior doctors, the resource was rolled out to NMPs. The core contents have expanded to include most clinical scenarios prescribers will encounter.

Many Trusts actively encourage the NMP as experts in their clinical to provide update sessions to other colleagues. From a governance and competency aspect, there is a requirement that all NMPs will complete an annual declaration of competency document which will state the areas of competency that individual NMP has. This competency document asks the NMP to confirm that they are compliant with the Royal Pharmaceutical Societies

Prescribing Competency Framework (2016), and they keep themselves up to date; there is a list of questions including awareness of policies and expectations of practice.

Colleagues are sent a reminder informing them that it is an annual requirement of the NMP policy to submit this data; therefore, if it is not sent through, they are in breach of the policy. If there was an error or incident and the annual declaration to prescribe document had not been sent through, then this would be taken into account.

As mentioned previously, there is an expectation that the prescribers within the Trust will adhere to 80% compliance with the local health economy prescribing formulary. The NMP lead in conjunction with pharmacy colleagues is responsible for the monitoring of compliance of this. Prescribers working within hospital in-patient settings will use hospital drug charts. These charts have medications dispensed against them by the pharmacy within the hospital setting, and some acute hospitals have outsourced their dispensaries in accordance with recommendations following Lord Carter's review (2016) into clinical pharmacy provision within secondary care. Hospital pharmacy departments will use electronic software programmes to review and audit prescribing patterns by individual prescribers.

The NMP lead will have oversight of this data as well as the data generated by analysing prescribing data from other sources. These may include a review of the electronic prescribing analysis and costs (ePACT) data generated from the data held by the NHS business services authority (NHSBSA) concerning the prescriptions known as FP10s used within primary care. This data is attributed to each prescriber though at times there may be inaccuracies due to processing errors, humans are involved and sometimes an error can occur especially with drugs which have very similar names. If there is a concern over this data, the NMP lead can request a copy of the FP10 held by the NHSBSA for assurance and governance purposes. The copy of the FP10 will either uphold or dispute the area of concern.

Other clinical areas may use different systems in which to audit prescribing activity. Her majesties prisons (HMP) prisons tend to use IT programmes such as SystmOne. The use of a single data system across the prisons reduces the possibility of errors as data is easily transferrable across multiple sites, and prisoners may be moved at short notice across the country; therefore, accurate easily transferrable data is essential.

Sexual health services will use a different software package to record their prescribing activity, and this data is anonymised in accordance with the requirements of the service. Prescribing decisions and the supply of medicines to either treat, or as part of contraceptive services, are recorded in this anonymised data sets. The NMP lead can request to see an overview of what was prescribed but not to whom attendees to the clinics are identifiable via a number only so as to protect the identity of the person attending the clinic. Trends of prescribing practice within the sexual health clinics can be determined from this anonymised data from the pharmacy department supplying the clinics compared to the data held on the software system.

Another important aspect of the NMP lead's role relates to the close working practices with the universities which provide NMP courses. As stakeholders we are key to providing feedback from the students we have supported their particular university but also with the professional bodies. The varying professional bodies whether that be the NMC, Healthcare professions council (HCPC) or General pharmaceutical council (GpHC) require the universities when they accredit and validate the courses to provide evidence of engagement with the local NMP leads. Regular meetings and the sharing of feedback between course leaders and the NMP leads enhance relationships between all concerned.

In conclusion, the role of the NMP lead is a core governance role providing strategic vision for developing NMPs for the future. There may be some variations in this role across different Trusts, but the core underlying principles remain the same, being governance, monitoring and support for non-medical prescribers within their Trust.

Self-assessment test

1   What is the definition of multidisciplinary care?
2   What is required for effective team working?
3   What is the role of the NMP lead in an NHS Trust?

Reflective exercise

You have now read through and studied the contents of this chapter, and it is time for you to reflect on what you have learnt and how you are going to relate this to your prescribing practice. From what you have learnt, consider how this will influence what you prescribe. Will the information that you have learnt change any of the prescribing decisions that you thought you may have had previously, and if so, what, how and why?

References

Department of Health. (2000). *A health service of all talents, developing the NHS workforce.* London: HMSO.

Department of Health. (2001). *Essence of care.* London: HMSO.

Department of Health. (2002). *Liberating the talents.* London: HMSO.

Lord Carter Review of Pharmacy Services. (2016). Available at https://www.pharmaceutical-journal.com/news-and-analysis/carter-review-calls-for-more-clinical-pharmacists-to-be-deployed-by-nhs-trusts/20200670.fullarticle?firstPass=false#fn_1.

Mitchell, G.K., Tieman, J.J., & Shelby-James, T.H. (2008). Multidisciplinary care planning and teamwork in primary care. *MJA.* 188(8), 563.

Royal College of Nursing. (RCN). (2012). Fact sheet: nurse prescribing in the UK. Available at https://www.rcn.org.uk/about-us/policy-briefings/pol-1512. Accessed 29 June 2020.

Afterword
Closing comments – the future of non-medical prescribing

Alison Pooler

We hope you have found this small companion book for non-medical prescribing a useful resource during your prescribing training. It has given you an overview of all the central features of any non-medical prescribing course in the UK, the content of which is governed by the Royal Pharmaceutical Society Competency Framework and guided by the professional bodies in their prescribing educational standards.

Non-medical prescribing has come a long way since its first introduction in community nurses and has expanded in the number of different health care professionals who can now train to become non-medical prescribers, thus enhancing the service and care delivery within the health service for increased outcomes for our patients and clients. This will expand further as pre-registration nursing students have increased pharmacological content within their curriculums to enable them to be prescribing ready upon graduation and which after a few years of clinical experience will be ready to take on further development to become a non-medical prescriber themselves, thus expanding the workforce further in prescribing rights to increase patient access and outcomes further, alongside our medical prescribing colleagues.

Index

adverse drug reactions 34; children 55; elderly 60; iatrogenesis 121–122; yellow card 36–37
antimicrobial resistance 117–120

bioavailability 20–21, 27; elderly 57
biomedical model 108–109
branded drug name 16

children 51–55; Childrens Act [1989] 95; Gillick competence 95
clinical management plan (CMP) 4, 7–9
compliance 60, 76, 108; elderly 56
consent 96–97
consultation models 71–74; Byrne and Long (1976) 72–73; Calgary-Cambridge communication skills framework 73–74; dysfunctional consultations 107; Neighbours model (1987) 71–72; Pendleton, Schofield, Tate and Havelock (1984) 4, 7–9
Crown Report (DH 1989, 1999) 2–3, 98
Cumberledge Report (DHSS 1986) 2

dependent prescribing 7
drug allergy/reactions 34–36

drug development 32–33
drug formulation 19, 21
drug interactions 25, 33–34, 50
drug licensing 31, 53
drug misuse and abuse 120–121

elderly 25, 40–41, 56–61
enzyme processes 24, 29, 46–47, 58
ethical aspects 93–98
extended formulary 2

first pass metabolism 20, 57

generic drug name 16

half life 26, 45
health beliefs 103–104, 107, 112
history taking 74–78; clinical decision making 78, 106; SOCRATES 75; SWIFT 105–106; TROCARSS 106

Independent prescribing 3, 9; paramedics 4; physiotherapists 4; podiatrists 4; scope of practice/competence 4, 10; in supplementary prescribing 7; therapeutic radiographers 4

legal aspects 84–92; *Bawa-Garba v GMC* [2018] 92; *Bolam v Friern Hospital Management Committee* [1957] 90; *Bolitho v City and Hackney Health Authority* [1998] 91; controlled drugs 87–88; *Donoghue v Stevenson* [1932] 90; *Gillick v West Norfolk and Wisbech Area Health Authority* [1985] 95; Human Medicines Regulation (2012) 86; Medicines Act (1968) 86; Misuse of Drugs Act (1971) 86, 88; Misuse of Drugs Regulation (2001) 86, 88; *R v Bawa-Garba* [2015] 92
liver disease 25, 45–51, 59
locus of control 103–104, 107

Mental Capacity Act (2005) 94, 96–97
multidisciplinary working (MDT) 122, 137–139

non-medical prescribing leads 139–144

Offences Against the Persons Act (1861) 96

patient access 2, 5
pharmacodynamics 27; enzyme processes (*see separate item*); receptors 27–29; transporter systems 30–31
pharmacokinetics 19; absorption 19–22, 44, 52, 61; distribution 19, 22, 44, 52, 61; elimination 19, 25–26, 45, 47, 52, 61; metabolism 19, 24, 44, 46, 52, 61
polypharmacy 33
pregnancy 61–65; breast feeding 65; drug effects 63–65; tetragenesis 62–64
prescription errors 6
prescription writing: BNF usage 126–127; children 54; cost effectiveness 132–135; influences 110–111; legal aspects 86–87; practical aspects 128–131; reasons for 109–110; repeat prescriptions 131–132; types of prescription 128
professional aspects of prescribing 82–84; accountability 82–84; professional regulators 83–84
public health 116–117, 123

renal insufficiency/disease 23, 26, 34, 41–45, 50, 59
routes of administration 17–20, 27, 53
Royal Pharmaceutical Society Competency Framework 10, 74

sociological models of health 108
supplementary prescribing 4, 7, 69; dieticians 4; pharmacists 4; physiotherapists 4; podiatrists 4

Printed in the United States
By Bookmasters